C000070385

THE
CANCER
SOLUTION

The revolutionary, scientifically proven program for the prevention and treatment of cancer

Robert O. Young
Matt Traverso

Library of Congress Cataloging-in-Publication Data

Young, Robert; Traverso, Matt
The Cancer Solution
Manufactured in the United States of America
ISBN 9781797964409

«The great enemy of truth is very often not the lie—deliberate, contrived and dishonest—but the myth—persistent, persuasive and unrealistic. Too often we hold fast to the clichés of our forebears. We subject all facts to a prefabricated set of interpretations. We enjoy the comfort of opinion without the discomfort of thought.»

—John F. Kennedy

Sir William Osler – one of the greatest medical icons and widely referred to as the Father of Modern Medicine – was chief physician of the John Hopkins Hospital and co-founder of the John Hopkins School of Medicine. He created the first residency program for specialty training for physicians and was the first to bring medical students out of the lecture halls and to the patients bedside. One day, while he was training doctors on how to best help their patients, he said:

«One of the first duties of the physician
Is to educate the masses not to take medicine.»

—Sir William Osler
Father of Modern Medicine
(https://it.wikipedia.org/wiki/William_Osler)

DISCLAIMER

The information contained in this book is for informational and educational purposes only. These statements have not been evaluated by the Food and Drug Administration.

This material is written for the express purpose of sharing educational information and scientific research gathered from the studies and experiences of the authors, healthcare professionals, scientists, nutritionists and informed health advocates.

Before beginning any practice relating to health, diet or exercise, it is highly recommended that you first obtain the consent and advice of a licensed health care professional.

The information contained herein is not intended to replace a one-on-one relationship with a doctor or qualified health care professional. Therefore, the reader should be made aware that this information is not intended as medical advice, but rather a sharing of knowledge and information from the research and experience of the authors.

The publisher and the authors encourage you to make your own health care decisions based upon your research and in partnership with a qualified health care professional. You and only you are responsible if you choose to do anything based on what you read.

PRAISE FOR *THE CANCER SOLUTION*

"*The Cancer Solution* by Dr. Robert Young and Matt Traverso is one of the most important books you will ever read. I am delighted to recommend this wonderful resource to anyone who wants to take control of their health and prevent or even reverse cancer."
—John P. Salerno, MD, World renowned medical authority on anti-aging and weight loss

"This book is a MUST read for anyone interested in creating vibrant health and a sustainable nutritional program for a healthy body. Many have healed from life threatening illnesses such as cancer just by making the fundamental changes in their diets and implementing the powerful tools offered in this groundbreaking book. This inspiring, life-changing book is an easy read that makes so much common sense, yet it is backed up with countless scientific studies and undeniable proof, all of which will inspire you to take your health into your own hands. I recommend reading it from cover to cover and then taking its principles into your life, to promote general health and wellbeing and increased energy levels. Your body will thank you!"
—Brandon Bays, Author, Founder, TheJourney.com

"Controlling the body's systemic pH balance during a person's life, using either an alkalinizing diet and/or buffering strategies, may help a lot in preventing the vast majority of diseases, including cancer. By the same token therapies based on alkalization may help in curing or at least stabilizing many incurable diseases, including a global nightmare such as cancer today. This book will help in understanding more on this issue."
—Stefano Fais, MD, PhD, Head Anti-Tumor Drug Section, The National Institute of Health

"At last—here are practical, effective steps on how to fight cancer and win."
—Elisabetta Macorsini, PhD, Biologist, Scientific Consul for Human Nutrition for The National Board of Biologists

"New research validates Dr. Young's findings on the true cause of cancer. This book provides the definitive answer to the cause, prevention and cure of cancer and of a great many diseases that plague the world today."
—Emanuele Ugo D'Abramo, MD, World Renowned Medical Doctor

"With the knowledge of *The Cancer Solution* in your hands you can change your destiny, you can cancer-proof your body and escape the devastation of medical intervention."
—Roy Martina, MD, World Renowned Medical Doctor

"This wonderful book will show you how, by adopting an alkaline diet and lifestyle, you can regain your natural inner balance at a cellular level and create optimal health. I hope this book will be translated in all languages to make this lifesaving information accessible to everyone in the world."
—Prof. Angelo De Giglio, University of Chemistry

"The Cancer Solution is the fastest way to lose weight, prevent disease, restore health, and feel better than ever."
—Stefano DiVecchio, MD

CLIENTS' TESTIMONIALS

Hodgkin's Lymphoma Cancer Reversed In 3 Months

My name is Ingrit Vaher. I am 31 years old and I have experienced something amazingly beautiful. It completely changed my perception towards my life and my health.

In December 2008 I was diagnosed to have Hodgkin's disease (lymph cancer), which had already developed to the second stage. My doctor recommended that I start a five month long chemotherapy treatment immediately and continue after that with radiation treatment. As per the doctor this was the only possible treatment for this aggressive disease.

Knowing about the disease shocked me, even though a part of me wasn't surprised at all. During my life I had already suffered from sugar addiction, gradually increasing weight, sleep and eating disorder and mood changes. Additionally, during my adulthood I suffered from strong depression, which I wasn't able to beat even after several attempts. I hated myself for it and I didn't appreciate my life.

After the diagnosis I felt great compassion towards my body. I remembered stories about people recovering from "incurable" diseases. I knew that I wanted to try the same. I decided not to start chemotherapy, at least for now. I believe that the mind and the emotions can effect the body and it is this belief that gave me courage. I knew that I was responsible for my sickness and I hoped that I could also heal it myself.

Luckily I had already read Dr. Robert O. Young's book and learned about pH balance theory. Immediately after the diagnosis I went for live blood microscopy. When I saw the microscopic pictures of my blood cells I decided to start the 21-day-long purification treatment using Innerlight products, developed by Dr. Robert O. Young. During the first week I was worried and afraid that the tumors in my throat were growing too fast, which would mean that I wouldn't have time to see the effects of the treatment and I would have to go for chemotherapy or surgery anyway.

During the second week the worst symptoms such as weakness, vomiting feeling etc. were away giving me more hope. During the third week I felt so much better that I knew I would heal by natural means without chemotherapy. Frankly, during the third week I felt better than ever in my adult life. The sugar addiction and the sleep disorder that had lasted for years were over. Despite the gloomy circumstances I felt very well-balanced, happy and grateful. At that point my friends started asking me the reason for my beautiful and healthy looks.

Three months after the diagnosis I asked for a whole-body scan. The doctors were surprised to see that the cancer was gone! Of all the tumors only two little dots remained. Of course I knew this because of how I felt, but still it made me tremendously happy to know that my recovery was so fast.

Throughout my life I've got to know different kinds of diets and natural products. The alkaline way of life and the Innerlight products are the only ones that helped me get rid of all my ailments including cancer. I'm grateful to Dr. Young for giving me new life, which I am happy leading in an alkaline way.

Richard Adgo's pH Miracle Story

I would like to share with you my story as to how I became involved with the pH Miracle Living Center in Valley Center, California, owned and operated by Dr. Robert O. Young.

In January, 2003, my osteopath noticed a mole change on my back. It was bleeding so he suggested that I should see my GP as soon as possible, like the next day. This I did and my GP took the mole out and sent it away for a biopsy. Two days later I received a phone call from my GP asking me to come and see him as soon as possible. This I did. My GP told me that the biopsy proved malignant, suggesting that I should make an appointment to see a plastic surgeon.

My wife and I went to see the surgeon about three days later and I was told that I had melanoma—a very invasive form of cancer. Given a ratio of between one and three I had number two. The doctor recommended that I have surgery as soon as possible, which I did. After surgery I was told I would have to have three monthly checkups

v

to make sure the cancer was not spreading. About four months later I felt a lump under my left armpit about the size of a marble, so I returned to the surgeon to find out that I would have to have my lymph nodes out. A week later I had the surgery and the doctor recommended me to the oncology department.

At this point I had met a lot of people with this condition and the outlook was not very bright. It was then that I decided to take charge of my own health.

I would like to share something with you at this point. My wife had bought Dr. Young's book Sick and Tired. I use to see it around a lot and it got to me so much that I would keep turning it over so that I could not see it. Strange as it may seem, that's how depressed I was. I couldn't see the wood for the trees. Very soon after that, Karen, my wife, booked both of us on a flight to the U.S where I attended a pH Miracle Living Retreat at the pH Miracle Living Center, in Valley Center, California. It was a five day Retreat and it was full on from day one, learning and understanding the New Biology(R). After only a few days I started to feel a lot better, with more energy and a lot less tired. I had not fallen asleep at all during the day even through all the lectures. I was on my way up. What a great feeling. But a major change in diet and a complete lifestyle change was ahead of me. Dr. Young said that he had given me the tools to look after myself and it was up to me now to make it happen.

It has been over six years now and I have never felt so good in all my life. I very rarely get anything like a cold or a flu, aching joints, headaches, or feel depressed. The pH Miracle is exactly what it says it is, just that. Thank you Dr. Young. I feel that with the help of all the people like my wife and my GP, my surgeon and Dr. Young I am still around to share this story with you. So really do not close off any doors when you are in such a situation. Take all the avenues and most of all take charge of your own health. Do not be told by anyone that you can go home and get things in order, which in other words means go home and die. Do what I have done and believe in the New Biology(R). Just get on with life. Make those lifestyle and dietary changes and just get on the Young pHorever pH Miracle program and give it your best and honest shot. Do not blame someone else for your condition, just get on with it. As I have. Become a pH Miracle all for the sake of trying. It's as simple as that. Get on the Doc Broc Greens and the pHour salts, and the pHlavor salts and the pHlush salts and the puripHy salts. It is called the COWS pack and you can order it at:

http://www.phmiracleliving.com/p-383-young-phorever-cows-starter-pack.aspx

All the best and have an alkaline pH Miracle day,

Richard Adgo
New Zealand

PS I would highly recommend you go to a pH Miracle Living Retreat. It will change your life and save your life. To sign up for the next Retreat in your area go to:

Szilvia Kovacs Cancer Reversal

Hello! I am Szilvia Kovacs from Hungary and I would like to thank Dr. Young, the father and developer of the pH Miracle.

I was diagnosed with a tumor in September 2008, then I had an operation and underwent long treatments.

After all this my doctors and some alternative practitioners basically gave up on me. They said I would probably die within a relatively short period of time and that I would be suffering up until the end.

My doctor, who did all he could, encountered things in my case that he could not really do anything about. Although since 2008 he was doing a lot, there were things he was not able to change at all.

Then I decided that after trying countless methods I give myself one more chance to my health, myself and my life. I chose life and I said yes to it. So I contacted Dr. Young in March 2010 and we met for one week. He showed me the method he uses to heal and did treatments on me.

After arriving home I continued them with incredible results. I received the first treatment on the 29th of March and did it for two more weeks at home. I had a test on the 4th of May and all my tests were good, the results were all negative!

I feel fantastic! I need very little time for rest. Foods have changed, finally I can really taste them! My thoughts are clearer and I am much calmer and more balanced. I can thank all this to alkalizing. I must say that all my life and everything has changed around me.

Thank you!

Cindy Wheatcraft pH Miracle Breast Cancer Testimonial

On April 9th, 2009 I was diagnosed with Ductal Cell Carcinoma of the right breast. The medical doctors found it in a routine mammogram. I had no symptoms and could not feel the lump until they pointed it out to me. I had not been feeling well for a couple of years though.

I was only 47 years old when I was diagnosed and had been thinking that my metabolism was just slowing down. I was also struggling with heavy blood flow during my menstrual cycle, which they told me was due to 2 large fibroid tumors and anemia. I have also been dealing with Irritable Bowel Syndrome for most of my life after being diagnosed in 1999. At times I have been disabled from this condition.

I own a Healing Center in Ohio and I started working with a Tom Frazier who had been studying Dr. Young's work for around 10 years. He came to work with me about a year and half before my diagnosis, so I have been learning about Dr. Young and the work he was doing.

I started out playing around with the Dr. Young's pH Miracle diet. I was also saying to myself, "I wonder what it will take for me to do this lifestyle and diet 100%." Watch what you say to yourself

Just before starting the pH Miracle lifestyle and diet 100% I found out that there was something remarkable on a routine mammogram that needed to be checked into. I was advised to have a digital mammogram. They showed me a mass in my right breast on the x-ray. The Doctor then did an Ultra Sound, and I could tell that something alarmed her. She called in the radiologist and I could tell by his face that I had cancer. They did a needle biopsy. That all happened on a Thursday.

When I suspected that I had a very aggressive breast cancer with very low survival rates, I immediately started doing research so when I got the official results on Monday I would be ready. The Doctors called me on Monday and gave me the bad news. I was diagnosed with

Ductal Cell Carcinoma—a very aggressive, fast growing/fast spreading cancer. The breast cancer surgeon said that I needed to have the mass taken out along with some lymph nodes. The oncologist said that I need follow-up radiation and chemotherapy for at least 5 years.

After much prayer, soul searching, meditation, contemplation and research I decided not to have the cancerous mass or the lymph nodes taken out. I also decided not to undergo the radiation or chemotherapy. I decided that I was going to follow Dr. Young's pH Miracle alkaline lifestyle and diet 100% from the pH Miracle book.

I officially started on the pH Miracle diet on April 13th. I found out on August 28th that I was cancer free! That's right! No tumor or mass or inflammation of the breast or the lymph nodes.

I saw Dr. Young in June when he came to New York City during a 2-day pH Miracle Retreat. He did a live and dried blood cell analysis and saw the cancerous breast condition and also saw that this cancerous condition started in my body 15 years before. I immediately started thinking back to what had happened to me 15 years earlier. That was when I got divorced, which was a very traumatic event in my life! I was totally amazed that Dr. Young could see physical and emotional stressors in my body from 1 drop of blood.

Dr. Young also told me that I needed to switch to a "Juice Feast" for 12 to 16 weeks. I started only drinking juiced green electron-rich alkaline vegetables and blended vegetables (energy soup). It was not easy at first, but then my body and mind shifted and started thriving on this live, electron-rich, alkaline food. My IBS, that I had suffered with for years went away immediately and completely.

My menstrual bleeding has lessened and is more normal, so I have noticed that my fibroids are healing.

My Mom and my son Tyler are doing the pH Miracle lifestyle and diet with me too. People are coming up to us all of the time saying "what are you 3 doing, you are all glowing." People have been commenting to me routinely about how great I look, how my eyes are sparkling, and how young I am looking. This diet is truly the diet for anti-aging!

On August 21st I went for a Thermography Test (Thermal Imaging) of my breasts. They sent the results to the doctors at Duke University and it came back that I no longer had Ductal Cell Carcinoma breast cancer in my right breast. When they did the needle biopsy of the tumor they left a titanium marker in the tumor. The Thermal Imaging detected the titanium marker but there was no cancer tumor around the marker or anywhere else in my right breast or upper part of my body. The tumor vanished! It was gone for good!

I have not felt this good in years, and actually, I have never felt this good! As a child, I was always complaining of "stomach aches".

Thank you Dr. Young! Your expertise, your life's work and the time you spent with me saved my life!

Cindy Wheatcraft
Hiram, Ohio
cindylee761@wheatcraft.net
216-346-1894

CONTENTS

INTRODUCTION

Dear Friend,

If you are reading these lines right now… you are blessed!

I (Matt) cannot express how excited I am to present this information to you. My purpose and mission in life is to help create a whole new paradigm of health, happiness and freedom!

The information you're about to read in this book has the power to ABSOLUTELY TRANSFORM your life in a way you have never imagined, or conceived possible.

It has helped turn cancer terminal patients (people labelled "soon to be dead" with no hope) into lively, thriving, and healthy individuals.

Because despite what doctors and the pharmaceutical and health care industries would have you believe, there is now a simple, easy and natural way to control, manage and actually *cure* cancer from your life and those you love. This breakthrough methodology, developed by world renowned scientist Dr Robert O. Young, has been a long time coming, and has already been used successfully for thousands and thousands of cancer patients.

Now in case you're skeptical, please know this, the real reason most doctors tell you that little can be done for your cancer, other than a horrible life of medicine and suffering, is PROFIT. That's right, it's more profitable for the medical industry to keep you sick and medicine dependent than to cure you, and that's a very sad fact to say the least. Corruption in medicine runs more rampant today than any other time in history.

> "Everyone should know that the "War on Cancer" is largely a fraud."
> —Linus Pauling PhD (Two Time Nobel Prize Winner, Author of several books on Vitamin C and cancer).

> "Conventional cancer treatments are in place as the law of the land because they pay, not heal, the best."
> —John Diamond, M.D. & Lee Cowden, M.D.

1

"For those of you who have lost loved ones to cancer know that when you support charities sponsored by the ACS you are unknowingly supporting the very drug companies who denied your loved ones any treatment except those that have already been proven to fail. According to the FDA *'Only a drug can cure, prevent or treat a disease'* but that is a lie! 'There have been many Cancer Cures, and all have been ruthlessly and systematically suppressed with Gestapo-like thoroughness by Cancer establishments"
—Robert C. Atkins, M.D.

"Most cancer patients in this country die of chemotherapy. Chemotherapy does not eliminate breast, colon, or lung cancers. This fact has been documented for over a decade, yet doctors still use chemotherapy for these tumors... Women with breast cancer are likely to die faster with chemo than without it."
—Allen Levin, MD UCSF

"My studies have proved conclusively that untreated cancer victims live up to four times longer than treated individuals. If one has cancer and opts to do nothing at all, he will live longer and feel better than if he undergoes radiation, chemotherapy or surgery."
—Professor Hardin B. Jones, Ph.D.

"More people live off cancer than die from it."
—Dr. Deepak Chopra, M.D.

"What if cancer is a systemic, chronic, metabolic disease of which lumps and bumps constitute only symptoms? Will this not mean that billions of dollars have been misspent and that the basic premises on which cancer treatment and research are grounded are wrong? Of course it will, and in decades to come a perplexed future generation will look back in amazement on how current medicine approached cancer with the cobalt machine, the surgical knife, and the introduction of poisons into the system and wonder if such brutality really occurred."
—Dr. Harold W. Harper, M.D.

It's a sad fact that the pharmaceutical and medical organizations lie to you to protect the status quo... and because of this you never learn the truth about cancer, and worse, its prevention. The truth that 99% of all people are not aware of is that cancer can actually be stopped before it ever enters your life! And better still, cancer can even be *reversed* without so much as taking a single pill or any medicine whatsoever!

REMEMBER CANCER IS NOT A DEATH SENTENCE , THE WRONG TREATMENT IS!

"A study of over 10,000 patients shows clearly that chemo's supposedly strong track record with Hodgkin's disease (lymphoma) is actually a lie. Patients who underwent chemo were 14 times more likely to develop leukemia and 6 times more likely to develop cancers of the bones, joints, and soft tissues than those patients who did not undergo chemotherapy (National Cancer Institute Journal 87:10)."
—John Diamond, M.D.

"Success of most chemotherapy is appalling...There is no scientific evidence for its ability to extend in any appreciable way the lives of patients suffering from the most common organic cancer... Chemotherapy for malignancies too advanced for surgery which accounts for 80% of all cancers is a scientific wasteland."
—Dr Ulrich Abel, M.D.

"Most cancer patients in this country die of chemotherapy. Chemotherapy does not eliminate breast, colon or lung cancers. This fact has been documented for over a decade, yet doctors still use chemotherapy for these tumours...Women with breast cancer are likely to die faster with chemo than without it."
—Alan Levin, M.D.

"Finding a cure for cancer is absolutely contraindicated by the profits of the cancer industry's chemotherapy, radiation, and surgery cash trough."
—John Diamond, M.D.

"We have a multi-billion dollar industry that is killing people right and left, just for financial gain. Their idea of research is to see whether two doses of this poison is better than three doses of that poison."
—Glen Warner, M.D. Oncologist

3

"As a chemist trained to interpret data, it is incomprehensible to me that physicians can ignore the clear evidence that chemotherapy does much, much more harm than good."
—Alan Nixon, Ph.D., Past President, American Chemical Society.

In the pages that follow I have presented practical, proven step-by-step methods for seizing (for yourself and your family) optimum health and TOTALLY FREE YOURSELF from disease and from the fear of ever getting ill or sick in the first place.

A lot of the information I'm about to share with you will fly in the face of what the medical establishment preaches. But understand, just because the majority believe something does not make it true. All the information here is based upon sound scientific studies. Dr. Robert O. Young, clearly the leading nutritional microbiologist in the world today, has been researching this field for over 25 years, with extraordinary results.

Therefore my goal at this moment is to deliver this information to you in an easy to understand way, but also in a way that will have tremendous impact on you, so you remember it, and USE it to change your life. For what good is inspiration if it's not backed up by *action*?

So strap on your seatbelt. "Empty the cup." And get ready to see your life transform faster than you ever thought possible!

YOUR GREATEST TREASURE

Stop and think for a second about how magnificent the workings of your body truly are...

Without you even having to think about it, and despite all the demands you make of it, your body produces billions of new cells every second, makes you hear, feel, see, smell, taste... regulates your temperature... operates this incredibly powerful super-computer called your brain...

Your body is the result of billions of years of evolutionary perfection. It puts any man-made technology to shame.

It is a beautifully created, perfectly and delicately balanced self-healing organism.

And yet most of us take this miracle completely for GRANTED!

Worst, still... we abuse it!

Know this: you ALWAYS end up paying the price (or reaping the rewards) for your life choices.

HONOR your body. RESPECT it. Your body is your VESSEL OF LIFE.

To NOT take care of your body is to reject LIFE.

Every moment of your life you have a CHOICE—what you put in your mouth, whether to exercise or not, whether to smoke, take drugs, drink alcohol, eat meat... or not.

Vibrant Health or Pain & Disease, you will soon discover, is a CHOICE.

Please, choose wisely.

THE CURRENT DISEASE EPIDEMIC—
REACHING CRISIS POINT

Despite major advances in science and technology, the human race has never been so diseased.

- 1 in 3 Americans will die of Cancer. *[National Center for Health Statistics]*
- 1 in 2 Americans will die of Heart Disease. *[National Center for Health Statistics]*
- 21 million Americans are diagnosed with Diabetes (35% of the population has Diabetes, but has not been diagnosed yet). *[Center for Disease Control (CDC)]*
- 43 million Americans suffer from Arthritis.). *[Center for Disease Control (CDC)]*
- Autoimmune Diseases affect 1 out of 5 people in U.S.A. *[American Autoimmune Related Disease Association]*
- Osteoporosis affects 28 million Americans. *[American Academy of Orthopaedic Surgeons]*
- 64% of the American population is overweight. *[Center for Disease Control (CDC)]*
- 42 million people in the world currently live with AIDS. *[World Health Organization (WHO)]*
- 121 million people worldwide suffer from Depression. *[World Health Organization (WHO)]*

95% of Americans will die of either Heart Disease, Cancer, or Diabetes (these are preventable, lifestyle-related and diet-related diseases, by the way).

If you are reading this right now and you lead the same lifestyle as the average person, THAT is your most probable outcome.

Despite billions of dollars being spent on discovering drugs for cancer, ironically, cancer has gone from being the #7 cause of death in 1970 in the US to the #2 cause currently. A child under the age of three has a 1 in 2 chance of developing cancer in its lifetime.

And at the same time the cost of health care is getting **bigger** and we as a society continue to get *sicker*.

Yes, it's a sad fact that despite massive expenditures on medical treatments and drugs, Americans are sicker than ever before in our history. One might wonder why the so-called "miracle drugs" manufactured and promoted by pharmaceutical companies—not to mention the highly touted medical "breakthroughs"—have neither prevented nor cured disease in this country.

The answer is this: Disease is big business.

In 2007, total national health expenditures rose 6.9%—two times the rate of inflation *(Health Affairs)*. The cost of treating patients reached an astronomical $2.7 TRILLION in 2011 *(CNN)*. U.S. health care spending is expected to reach $4.2 TRILLION in 2016, or 20% of GDP *(The National Coalition on Health Care)*.

And what's the result? More people are getting sicker today than ever before!!

One hundred years ago heart disease, cancer, and diabetes were virtually unknown. The increasing prominence of degenerative disease parallels the development of scientific medicine in the 20th century. In 1910 deaths from heart disease, diabetes and cancer were less than 10 percent of total deaths. **By 1997 more than 90 percent of the population was dying of these three diseases.** That's right, after 100 years of advances and breakthroughs in scientific medicine, the sad truth is that TODAY **these three diseases claim someone's life _every single second_.**

And, ironically, today we have MORE doctors, we have MORE hospitals, and we have *infinitely* MORE pharmaceutical drugs. *And what do we have to show for it?* The sickliest generation in American history!

This situation is quite simply horrific, and utterly unsustainable.

Since the '70s, the US has spent more on fighting cancer than on anything else except landing a man on the moon.

Despite spending more on health care per capita than any other country in the world, the United States are rated only 37th in the world in "overall health system performance" by the World Health Organization.

WHAT'S GOING ON?

WE HAVE AN EPIDEMIC ON OUR HANDS!
WHY ISN'T ANYONE SAYING ANYTHING ABOUT THIS??!
WHY DON'T WE HEAR ABOUT THIS EVERY DAY ON THE
NEWS???

*I believe the definition of insanity is doing the same over and over
and over and expecting a different result.*

*So what's really causing all this? What happened then over the last
century?*

THE BIGGER PICTURE

As I mentioned previously, <u>your body is the result of millions of years of evolutionary perfection</u>. It is a beautifully created, perfectly and delicately balanced self-healing organism.

OUR BODY : THE "2-MILLION YEAR-OLD CAR" METAPHOR

Imagine if you will that you are driving a 2-million year old car. An all-natural, organic, living, breathing car…

For 2 million years, this car has been using fuel such as:
water / seeds / nuts / grasses / herbs / roots / fruits / vegetables / cereals (uncooked, by the way—not processed until all their natural goodness is totally and utterly destroyed…)

THAT'S the fuel it is used to.

MOREOVER, THAT'S the fuel its entire system is based upon. It was MADE from that stuff.

Then, suddenly, after 2,000,000 years… that car switched over to—for the last 100 years—a new, modern mixture of:

sugar / sweets / biscuits / crisps / chocolate / coffee, tea, coca-cola / fats & oils / cigarettes / alcohol / vinegar / pharmaceutical drugs / caffeine / chemicals, pesticides, and preservatives (loads of them) / meat (loads of it) / milk, cheese, ice-cream / refined carbohydrates with ZERO nutritional value (white rice, white flour, white sugar, pasta, bread…) etc.

What do you think would happen to this 'vehicle'?

THAT'S RIGHT—**IT WOULD BREAK DOWN.**

So you bring it to the mechanic, right?

Now, is it in the mechanic's interest to resolve the SOURCE of the problem (your choice of fuel)?

Or does he give you the instant fix that you want to get the car going again for a little bit?

After all, you are a busy person, you've got places to go, you're experiencing pain and are 'immobilized', you need this problem <u>fixed</u> as soon as possible. You even ask for a 'fix'.

So… that's what the mechanic offers you.

A 'fix'.

Better yet: an INSTANT 'fix'.

(It's not going to last, mind you…)

Think about this carefully. WHAT SHOULD YOU DO?

What is the INTELLIGENT thing to do?

Keep taking the car to the mechanic, or clean the fuel tank and use a cleaner fuel?

For every health challenge out there, all you ever hear in the media or from doctors (the 'mechanic') is: *take this drug or that drug.*

Simply go to Dr. FeelGood & pop a pill to make yourself feel all better again…

Sure… take drugs to make the symptom go away...

But what about the SOURCE of the problem?

THE "MOSQUITO & STALE POND" METAPHOR

If you kill all the mosquitoes around a stale pond with DDT chemicals, you won't have mosquitoes for a little while.

But since the <u>SOURCE</u> of the problem is still there—the stale, disgusting pond where mosquitoes can find food and a propitious ground for laying their eggs—*mosquitoes will come back!*

It's the same with your body!

You need to eradicate THE SOURCE, THE ROOT of your health problems.

You see, ultimately, any ailment you experience comes from a breakdown within your body.

Diseases are just warning signs of something very fundamental happening inside of you—something is out of kilter. Something is unbalanced.

Deepak Chopra refers to this as "The *violation* of simple laws of nature that make our body function."

The richest — read: most industrialized, modern, far-from-natural — societies have the highest incidence of Cancer, Diabetes, Heart Disease, Arthritis, Osteoporosis, Multiple Sclerosis, Chronic Fatigue, Fibromyalgia, etc. despite the billions spent on so-called 'cures' by the pharmaceutical industry.

So… the most 'modern' societies are the sickliest on the planet.

Hmm. Interesting.

I wonder why.

THE TRUTH IS... YOU ARE OUT OF BALANCE

We now live a 'far-from-natural' lifestyle.

There are on average over 1500 synthetic industrial chemicals present in our bodies that did not exist 50 years ago. We are filled with toxins from the food, water, air, personal care products, and medication we ingest and use.

In as simple a language as possible, if the delicate balance of our body's systems are taken 'out of whack' because of our modern, unnatural lifestyle, we experience DISEASE.

Our diseases are nothing but a SYMPTOM of this imbalance.

If you adopt a healthy lifestyle (healthy diet & mindset, rest, exercise, cleanse & detoxify, etc.) you will put your body back into balance— that's what holistic medicine is all about.

The "holistic", "complimentary", "alternative" ways of treating people have been around for thousands of years, and they absolutely WORK.

Lead a healthy lifestyle and there is practically NO chance you'll ever suffer any of the ailments mentioned above.

What you will soon discover through these pages is that those ailments are all lifestyle and nutrition-related.

And yet you'll rarely hear this in the media. How come?

Here's the SHOCKING ANSWER...

11

BEWARE OF THE CULTURAL HYPNOSIS

"Let us first understand the facts, and then we may seek the cause"

—Aristotle

We live in a cultural hypnosis that has taught us that we are fragile.

We have been conditioned to believe that things are happening to us.

We have been **conditioned** to feel "in danger".

We have been **conditioned to believe** that drugs are the answer to disease.

I'm here to remind you of the truth… YOU ARE NOT FRAGILE.

The truth is that our natural state is one of Strength, Health, and Energy.

We are genetically programmed to be utterly HEALTHY and to THRIVE.

You are the end result of tens of thousands of generations of human beings, the pinnacle of evolutionary perfection. In fact, you are a genetic champion.

Most of us believe that our bodies are constantly under attack by bugs, germs, viruses…

Our society as a whole has been led to believe that most sickness and disease comes from external agents "attacking" our body.

This is simply not true.

The truth is that health comes from within, and is also lost from within.

The truth has been with us for thousands of years. It has been swept under the carpet, however, in the name of profit—it is in certain people's interest that we feel vulnerable.

You see, fear will make us buy and consume just about anything.

Keeping people afraid SELLS! It sells medicine. It sells newspapers. It increases TV news' ratings.

Television stations, radio stations, newspapers and magazines are paid billions in advertising to condition us a certain way. Do NOT believe ANYTHING the media tell you.

For example, every other week it seems that I hear on the news how this drug company or that drug company is just about to discover a cure for cancer.

Yup, the cure for cancer is just around the corner…

This charade has been going on for over 50 years! It is total manipulation.

BEHIND THE SCENES

*"The beginning of wisdom is to call
things by the right names."*
—Chinese Proverb

The root cause. That's where it all happens.

**Remember: your 'dis-ease' is a <u>symptom</u> of *<u>something very
fundamental</u>* happening within you.**

**Drugs deal with the short-term effect, the surface cause of your
discomfort, the <u>symptom</u>.** *Creating health and restoring your body
has **nothing**, and I repeat, **NOTHING** to do with drugs.*

**Make no mistake, the real <u>source</u> of the problem is the way you
live your life.**

It is a sad fact, but 99% of people out there are completely asleep.

Ignorant. Oblivious to what is really going on.

You see, conventional medicine (also known as orthodox or allopathic
medicine) utilizes poisonous substances (drugs) in non-lethal dosages
in order to suppress symptoms. *This approach neither addresses the
cause of the disease condition, nor is it responsible for healing the
patient.* Rather, the use of drugs will temporarily mask the
manifestations of the disease, while at the same time, drive the disease
deeper into the body...only to reappear at a later date, as a more
serious, and chronic health threat.

Do not assume that the only difference between allopathic and
alternative medicine, however, is an honest difference of opinion in the
philosophies on the origin of disease states. Hardly! There is, in truth, a
concerted agenda organized by the international pharmaceutical
companies *to suppress any and every alternative, non-drug therapy that
WORKS.*

Why?

Because they want people to keep on coming back for more treatments
and more drugs. A *cured* patient is a lost source of income (*cures kill
profits!*). A sick patient who is marginally "improved" is a *manageable*
patient.

14

Managing patients means routine office visits and renewing of drug prescriptions.

Therefore, a manageable patient is a *continuing source of income*; a cash cow if you will. Multiply that by a few hundred million people and you get an idea why this deceit is being put upon you. The profits from the so called "health-care" industry are *staggering!*

> Before we continue I want to make it clear that while **I support and believe in medical science**, I do not agree with the medical establishment and the pharmaceutical industry operating it that value profit and protection of the status quo over the health and wellness of the people.
>
> **Mainstream medicine is not going to the source of health problems. Doctors, as hard working and caring as they are, are primarily trained in the use of pharmaceuticals to treat illness.**

The thrust of the orthodox pharmaceutical agenda is to provide temporary relief, while never addressing the cause of the disease. This agenda insures regular visits to the doctor's office and requires the patient to routinely return to the pharmacy to refill his prescriptions.

This is what the game is all about folks, plain and simple.

There are a number of alternative approaches to health that work so well and cost so little (compared to conventional treatment) that the pharmaceutical industry is fighting tooth and nail to keep suppressed. The reason is obvious: Alternative, non-toxic therapies represent a potential loss of billions of dollars to the medical and drug companies.

> *"The individual is handicapped by coming face to face with a conspiracy so monstrous he cannot believe it exists."*
> —J. Edgar Hoover, ex-FBI Director

Through continuous marketing and advertising the public has been brainwashed into equating MEDICAL CARE with HEALTH, whereas in fact exactly the opposite applies: modern medicine has become the principal cause of disease today (Hans Ruesch).

Health journalist and author Nick Regush, well known for his masterful investigative reporting on health issues for CBC television, summed it up nicely: *"Medicine as we know it, is dying...The disease is caused by conflict of interest, tainted research, greed for big bucks, pretentious doctors and scientists, lying, cheating, invasion by the morally bankrupt marketing automatons of the drug industry, derelict politicians and federal and state regulators....As a journalist, it has become very plain to see how little anything the medical Establishment does these days can be trusted or taken at face value. Press conferences, journal articles, symposia—all are geared to spike and obfuscate the truth, to hide red flags from the public and to bulk up the shares of investors in the companies that are promoting the science and the researchers."*

In an unusually candid comment for a senior government official, Dr. Herbert Ley, former FDA commissioner, remarked:

> **"The thing that bugs me is that the people think the FDA is protecting them. It isn't. What the FDA is doing and what the public thinks it's doing are as different as night and day."**

You see, America's medical/industrial complex was organized around the American Medical Association, formed by drug interests for the purpose of manipulating the legal system.

Controlled by pharmaceutical companies, this complex has become a trillion-dollar-a-year business. It also includes many insurance companies, the Food and Drug Administration (FDA), hospitals, and university research facilities. All driven by drug companies.

Here's some interesting statistics about drug companies: The COMBINED PROFITS for the TEN most profitable drug companies in the Fortune 500 ($35.9 billion) are GREATER than the profits for all the other 490 companies *put together* ($33.7 billion)!!

Did you get that? I repeat: *The top ten pharmaceutical companies make more in profits than the rest of the Fortune 500 companies combined!!* And these 500 companies even include Microsoft and Apple! (By the way, the 'Fortune 500' is a ranking of the top most *profitable* American corporations.)

One could hope drug companies would decide to make some

RADICAL changes, but that is not what is happening. Instead, drug companies are doing more of what got them into this situation. *They are marketing their drugs even more relentlessly.* They are pushing even harder to extend their monopolies on top-selling drugs (prescription drug sales are *consistently rising well over 18% a year from previous years*). And they are pouring more money into lobbying and political campaigns.

In August 2004, Dr. Marcia Angell (an M.D.) published a very enlightening book entitled *"The Truth About The Drug Companies : How They Deceive Us and What To Do About It."* Dr. Angell's perspective is particularly interesting because for 20 years before her retirement in 2000, she was **executive editor and editor-in-chief of the New England Journal of Medicine,** one of the most prestigious medical journals in the world. Under her watch, the journal published **hundreds of studies** of new drugs. It also published blunt editorials harshly critical of the pharmaceutical industry and the way drugs are tested and approved in the United States. She makes several major points, in an interview published in the Los Angeles Times, which are critical for you to understand:

- *"Drugs are expensive, but not because of the costs of research. The money the largest drug companies spend on marketing and the amount of profit they make dwarfs their research expenditures. In 2002, for example, the biggest drug companies spent only about 14% of sales on research and development and 31% on what most of them call 'marketing and administration.' They consistently make more in profits than they spend on R & D. And their profits are immense. In 2002, the combined profits of the 10 drug companies in the Fortune 500 were $35.9 billion. That's more than the profits of the other 490 businesses put together, if you subtract losses from gains."*

- *"...the number of truly innovative new drugs is quite small. True, many drugs are coming to market. But most of them aren't new at all. They are minor variations of best-selling drugs that are already on the market."*

- *"Drug makers are only required to show that a new medication is more effective than a placebo, or sugar pill. If a drug works better than a placebo and is safe, the FDA approves it, and it can enter the market. The result is that doctors don't know if a new drug that comes along is any better or worse than the drugs they're already using."*

- *"...patents run out on older drugs and they can then be sold as generics at as little as 20% of the price (they sold at while still under patent). Pharmaceutical manufacturers need a constant supply of new drugs that have patent protection so they can charge whatever they want."*

- *"...why are drug companies spending so much on marketing? The answer is that they have to convince us that their me-too drugs are better than the others. And that takes a heap of marketing, because there's usually no scientific evidence to back up the claim."*

> *"Over the past two decades the pharmaceutical industry has moved very far from its original high purpose of discovering and producing useful new drugs. Now primarily a marketing machine to sell drugs of dubious benefit, this industry uses its wealth and power to co-opt every institution that might stand in its way, including the US Congress, the FDA, academic medical centers, and the medical profession itself."*
> —Dr. Marcia Angell, former Editor in Chief of The New England Journal of Medicine and a nationally recognised authority in the field of health policy and medical ethics

Please understand: Big Pharma (the pharmaceutical industry) isn't interested in finding cures for Cancer, AIDS, or Diabetes; to them, people who buy drugs are not patients...they are CUSTOMERS.

Customers make them profit. These huge pharmaceutical corporations are legally responsible for the increase in profit for them and their shareholders. Period.

If cancer is cured, they don't make profit. The drug companies would be out of business and the doctors would be out of jobs.

Corporations and other entities like the FDA know that **curing means the end of business.** *They can't make a living if you don't get sick.*

Big Pharma doesn't want a cure, they will NEVER discover a cure.

"Curing" people doesn't make any money. "Treatment" does. "Treatment" meaning treatment with drugs.

"Treatment" masks the symptoms of a problem. "Cure" means finding the cause of the problem and removing it. And drugs are designed to "Treat", not cure or prevent illnesses, where the patient becomes dependent upon them for life. With this "Treatment" idea forced upon us, as the only option we have available, we are being ripped off, and it's time we **woke up** and made better choices. Let's face it, long-term diseases—ones which sometimes mean a lifetime dependence on drugs, devices, medical interventions and treatments of all sorts—are among the most profitable revenue sources on the planet. For example, **cancer** is the quintessential disease that engenders lifelong dependency. More than many diseases, it illustrates the corporate model of modern sickness care that is keen on having you take products over and over and *over* again.

> *"This is the world that has been pulled over your eyes to blind you to the truth."*
> —Morpheus, in 'The Matrix'.

EVERYTHING YOU KNOW ABOUT HEALTH IS WRONG

Please wipe your slate clean of what you think you know about health. Most of what you know and think you know is misinformation. Let us together dismantle the myths of health that are killing us as a society.

We are lead to believe that germs and viruses cause disease.

And what should we do?

We should avoid or 'kill' the germs and maybe we can avoid the disease.

We are taught that illnesses like cancer and diabetes can just show up, for no good reason and that the only solution is medicine and surgery, if we're lucky that is.

We don't feel empowered about our health and we place it in the hands of experts and hope that when we get ill, they will be able to help us get healthy again and live longer.

After all we don't know what to do, so isn't it a good thing that we have all these experts and drugs researchers out there to tell us what to do?

Well let me ask you a question: How may 'wonder drugs' that we've been taught were supposed to make us healthier—have not worked? How many of these have been promoted to us by the so called "experts"?

Listen, the ultimate expert on your life is YOU by testing what works; not by looking around and being like everybody else.

If you do what everybody else does, you'll have what everybody else has—and do you know what that's like for the general population? It's not a pretty sight! One in two people dies of heart disease or diabetes! One in three dies of cancer!

We must think uniquely. We must think differently. We can't just accept what's being fed to everybody. We must become CRITICAL in our thinking!

And by the way, this is NOT an attack on the medical profession. **Doctors care so much!** They care immensely about human beings and they will give their heart and soul at the expense of their own health, emotions, or families to help other people recover from disease in the only way they know how.

We should feel compassion for doctors. Go and watch what a doctor has to do to make it through medical school. What a dehumanising process! It is unbelievable what they go through out of their desire to help others.

Medical school training is also an intentionally gruelling process, designed to physically push the weaker students over the edge.

They do this to make sure that as a doctor you will be able to take the pressure in a real life-or-death situation and that you won't trip up. Perhaps the intentions are good, but it's hardly a wholesome learning environment for the doctors!

Doctors in training are given more work than they could possibly do, and they learn early on to rely on all kinds of stimulants (i.e. chemicals) to stay up late to study.

Medical School is an abusive, destructive, dehumanising process. Students have zero time to stop and say: Hey, does this make ANY sense?

On top of all that, the half-life of the current medical education is 4 years. This means that a doctor leaving school today knows 50% more about medicine than someone who left 4 years ago. With so many patients to see, doctors rarely have time to further their education.

How do doctors keep 'up to date'?

So many new drugs come out every year—there's no way for doctors to keep up. Hence doctors are primarily educated about new advances in medicine by the drug companies' salesmen!

Of course, 70% of all drugs on the market today weren't even around 15 years ago. Someone has to educate them, and the pace at which all this is happening is amazing!

The Washington Post reports that a University of Washington study published in the Journal of the American Medical Association confirms the insidious influence drug advertising brings to bear on *perverting* American medicine. For many doctors, drug industry marketing is their **prime source of information**.

A series of studies have confirmed beyond a shadow of a doubt that doctors are influenced more by the advertising for the drug than by the scientific literature. However when doctors are confronted, they are usually unaware or unwilling to admit that they've been influenced by non-scientific sources.

A major reason why health care is in such a shambles is that the medical establishment has allowed itself to be bought off by the pharmaceutical industry.

The medical establishment works closely with the drug multinationals whose main objective is PROFITS, and whose worst nightmare would be an epidemic of good health.

An article in the Journal of the American Medical Association (JAMA) recently stated that oncologists (cancer doctors) make an average of $253,000 a year, of which 75% is profit from chemotherapy drugs administered in their offices.

These drugs are obscenely profitable, providing average profit margins of 30,000% to 50,000% over the cost of raw materials. Sometimes, their markups can be as high as 500,000% (yes you read that right, five hundred thousand percent), naturally drug companies will do anything to sell more pills.

To a pharmaceutical marketer, the doctor is the "first link in the chain of getting medication from manufacturer to consumer." Any physician can LEGALLY prescribe ANY medication for ANY use.

Obviously 100% of prescription drugs costs originate with a doctor's orders.

Doctors are rewarded with research grants, gifts, and lavish perks. The principal buyers are the public—from infants to the elderly—who MUST be *thoroughly medicated*...at any cost!

Physicians' choices *profoundly impact* sales of a drug company's products. So, pharmaceutical manufacturers focus their marketing budgets to *influence* those choices.

AN EPIDEMIC CAUSED BY PHARMACEUTICAL DRUGS

> "We don't need more medication; we need education."
> —Dr. Robert O. Young

A series of studies found that pharmaceutical drugs kill MORE people every year than are killed in traffic accidents.

Sadly the average 65 year old person in the United States takes an average of 11 medications a day! **More people take drugs today than ever before!**

In 2006, global spending on prescription drugs topped $643 billion, with the US accounting for almost half of the global pharmaceutical market. The US pharmaceutical industry is the most profitable of all businesses in the US.

And the irony is that there is not a single chronic disease which has been cured as a result of taking prescription drugs.

Despite the number of drugs available why are people sicker than ever? Drugs have not helped people, instead drug companies have made people addicted to drugs and suffering further from the side-effects of taking so many different combinations of drugs.

The *Journal of the American Medical Association* (the most prestigious of the American conventional medical journals and one of the most conservative) reported that an estimated 106,000 people die EACH YEAR from drugs which, by medical standards, are *properly* prescribed and *properly* administered. (JAMA, 1994, 272:23, p 1851. Also:

JAMA. 1998;279(15):1215-1216. Also: JAMA. 2000 Jul 5;284(1):95-7. Also: JAMA. 2000;284(4):483-485.) Again, these 106,000 deaths are NOT the result of physician errors; these are the result of *correctly* prescribed and *correctly* taken medical drugs.

Dr. Gary Null et al have published the most comprehensive and well-documented study reporting that *"The total number of iatrogenic deaths is 783,936. It is evident that the American medical system is the leading cause of death and injury in the United States."* [Life Extension. March, 2004]

The bottom line is the drug industry does NOT want people to get healthy. Because if everyone was healthy, *they wouldn't need to buy drugs*. The drug industry wants people to buy more drugs. Healthy people don't need drugs. If everyone was healthy, the drug industry would be out of business.

Remember, pharmaceutical companies have a fiduciary responsibility to their shareholders; AND THEIR LEGAL RESPONSIBILITY IS TO INCREASE PROFITS. And of course, drug companies earn profits from the *expansion* and *continuation* of disease (where patients are put on drugs for life).

The Cancer Industry

Consider that since 1971, when the "War on Cancer" started, about $2 trillion has been spent on conventional cancer treatment and research. Yet, despite the government and private sector's work to put a positive face on cancer survival rates, they <u>have not improved</u>. The latest statistics show more Americans dying from common cancers than ever before. For example, the January 10, 2002 issue of the New England Journal of Medicine stated that 20 years of clinical trials using chemotherapy on advanced lung cancer have yielded survival improvement of <u>only two months</u>.

In his interesting book World Without Cancer – The Story of Vitamin B17, G. Edward Griffin puts it this way: *"With billions of dollars spent each year in research, with additional billions taken in from the cancer-related sale of drugs, and with vote-hungry politicians promising ever-increasing government programs, we find that, today, there are more people making a living from cancer than dying from it.*

If the riddle were to be solved by a simple vitamin, this gigantic commercial and political industry could be wiped out overnight. The result is that the <u>science</u> of cancer therapy is not nearly as complicated as the <u>politics</u> of cancer therapy."

According to an article in the January, 2003 issue of *Life Extension, "the institutions we have counted on to find a cure (National Cancer Institute, American Cancer Society, drug companies, etc.) <u>have failed</u>. This is not an allegation, but an <u>admission</u> made by the National Cancer Institute itself."*

An interesting look at statistical evidence of the "success" of conventional cancer treatment was published in 2004 in the Journal of Clinical Oncology. This study looked at the records of over 200,000 patients with cancer in the U.S. and Australia from 1990 to 2004. The results of this study were astonishing, showing that chemotherapy has an average 5-year survival success rate of just over 2 percent for ALL cancers: **2.1%** in the U.S. and **2.3%** in Australia.

"And what about radiation?"

Radiation, although technically packaged, is equivalent to burning your cancer into extinction—it uses high-energy X-rays to kill cancer cells. The radiation does not distinguish between cancerous and non-cancerous cells and therefore the surrounding healthy cells are also destroyed. Cancer is a "systemic" condition. Your whole body is involved. Reducing the tumor size does not equate to curing the cancer.

Legislation claiming to protect the consumer from drugs is usually **written by** the drug industry. Politicians who are grateful for the financial support of the drug companies are eager to put their names on legislation and push for its enactment. Once it becomes law, it serves merely to **protect** the sponsoring drug companies against competition—from natural cancer treatments, for example. The consumer is **the victim** of this legislation, not the beneficiary.

In drug testing and marketing, unlike other industries that lobby Congress, there is the added necessity to pretend that everything is being done scientifically. Therefore, in addition to recruiting the aid of politicians, **scientists** must also be enlisted—a feat that is easily accomplished by the judicious allocation of funding for research.

This process is nothing new. Former FDA Commissioner James L. Goddard, in a **1966** speech before the Pharmaceutical Manufacturers Association, expressed concern about **dishonesty in testing** new drugs. He said:

"I have been shocked at the materials that come in. In addition to the problem of quality, there is the problem of dishonesty in the investigational new drug usage. I will admit there are gray areas in the IND [Investigation of New Drug] situation, but the conscious withholding of unfavorable animal clinical data is not a gray area. The deliberate choice of clinical investigators known to be more concerned about industry friendships than in developing good data is not a gray area."

Goddard's successor at the FDA was Dr. Herbert Ley. In 1969, he testified before the Senate committee and described several cases of **blatant dishonesty** in drug testing. One case involved an assistant professor of medicine who had tested **24 drugs for 9 different companies**. Dr. Ley said:

"Patients who died while on clinical trials were not reported to the sponsor... Dead people were listed as subjects of testing. People reported as subjects of testing were not in the hospital at the time of the tests. Patient consent forms bore dates indicating they were signed after the subjects died."

Another case involved a **commercial drug-testing firm** that had worked on 82 drugs from 28 companies. Dr. Ley continued:

"Patients who died, left the hospital, or dropped out of the study were replaced by other patients in the tests without notification in the records. Forty-one patients reported as participating in studies were dead or not in the hospital during the studies... Record-keeping, supervision and observation of the patients in general were grossly inadequate."

Shocking isn't it.

THE FACTS:

There are about 700,000 doctors in the US.

In the United States we're spending more on health care than ever before. And ironically the US leads the developed world in deaths from heart disease, prostate cancer, breast cancer, colorectal cancer, and diabetes.

The countries that use the most medicine are the most unhealthy. For example, the leading cause of death in our society today is modern medicine—*the healthcare system*—causing a total number of **783,936 deaths** per year. Just in the US. (Starfield, B. JAMA. 2000 (July 26): 284, 4. Also: Death by Medicine – Gary Null, PhD; Carolyn Dean MD, ND; Martin Feldman, MD; Debora Rasio, MD; and Dorothy Smith, PhD).

In 1968, America declared war on cancer. By February 1994, **the *Journal of the American Medical Association* declared the war on cancer a failure**. In all age groups, cancer incidence is increasing.

Adverse drug reactions are the # 4 cause of death in the United States.

So the very industry that is here to tell you, "We are providing your health," is causing an EPIDEMIC. That's **the leading cause of death in America.** And this is not Matt Traverso saying it. This is the American Medical Association Journal, 1994, 1998, and 2000.

> *"I firmly believe that if all the medicine in the world were thrown into the sea, it would be all the better for mankind—and all the worse for the fishes."*
> —Oliver Wendell Holmes, M. D.
> Professor Emeritus of Medicine at Harvard

The world is becoming sicker, fatter and more depressed than ever.

The good news is that the SOLUTION is in YOUR hands. It involves claiming your right to make your own decisions about your health.

There are *no "magic bullets"(drugs) when it comes to achieving good health.* Optimum health is the result of observing a series of simple natural laws—making right decisions day after beautiful day.

AN INVITATION

I (Matt) really want you to get everything you can out of this program. To do that, you'll have to change the way you think about health. Specifically, you must embrace the concept of **taking responsibility for your own health.**

Please understand: Your health is not some highly complex thing which you can't gain FULL CONTROL over. You don't have to hand over your health to an "expert" who will know what to do with it. All you need is the right information.

The absolute best person
to take charge of your health
is you.

A lot of the information that Dr. Young will share with you will seem RADICALLY different to what you've been taught in the past. That's fine, I totally respect that. You will have to decide what you're going to believe (though keep in mind that everything Dr. Young is sharing is backed up by 25 years of scientific research and extraordinary results with thousands and thousands of cancer patients).

But ultimately the best way to decide whether or not something is true is to try it and judge by the RESULTS in your own body.

If you do, I promise you a TOTAL TRANSFORMATION in your health and in the quality of your life beyond anything you ever thought possible.

Therefore our goal for this next part of this program is to empower you with breakthrough information to free yourself of cancer (or ANY disease for that matter) and create extraordinary energy in your life.

I am especially motivated to bring this lifesaving information to you since it appears that very few are daring enough to try to do so. And I can understand that. But my motivation is to help you get what we contract for: health care, and stop our *sick care.*

28

Again, I believe the definition of insanity is repeating the same process over and over again and expecting a different result. Chemotherapy, radiation and surgery as curative measures for cancer have failed miserably for the last 70 years and counting—without even mentioning the "quality" of life during the "treatment", if you know what I mean.

And still, I believe that there will be ever-increasing pressure to persuade patients to choose this insanity – driven by the illusion that this is their only source for a cure.

Please listen: The only person who can cure you is You. No doctor can eat your food, exercise your body, manage your thoughts and emotions and adopt a new lifestyle. Only you can do all of these things. Only you can fully understand and tune into your symptoms. Only you can DECIDE to triumph over cancer and reclaim your life.

We all must nurture, support and respect our immune system. Let's embrace life and live it to the fullest.

I trust this book will help you open your eyes, broaden your horizons, and find the solution that's already within you—in your body's miraculous self-healing ability to rebuild and repair itself.

> *I believe that wellness is your birthright, and my mission is to wipe out the false and contradicting health information that's plaguing the mainstream media. You're about to discover exactly how to cure cancer and transform your body into a healthy, energetic example of what life is supposed to be.*
>
> *Because the answers are always within us; found in our own immune systems and our own biology. We are living, breathing healing machines, and my task is to simply remind you of your true healing nature—and to show you how to take back your health power NOW!*

Please remember, it is your life; it is your health; and it is your choice. Choose wisely.

Let the enlightenment begin…

INTRODUCING DR. ROBERT O. YOUNG AND THE "PH MIRACLE"

I am very excited to introduce you to the work of the leading nutritional microbiologist in the world today—Dr. Robert O. Young.

Over the past two and a half decades, Dr. Young has been widely recognized as one of the top research scientists in the world. Throughout his career, his research has been focused at the cellular level. Having a specialty in cellular nutrition, Dr. Young has devoted his life to researching the true causes of "disease," subsequently developing The New Biology™ to help people balance their life.

THE NEW BIOLOGY

Dr. Young's scientific findings have led him to a new science he calls *The New Biology*^{TM}.

In contrast, the 'old' biology (based on the work of Louis Pasteur in the late 1800s) stems from the idea that disease comes from germs and bacteria which invade the body from the outside.

Simply put, the New Biology^{TM} states that there is only *One Sickness and One Disease*, and that this one 'sickness' is the over-acidification of the body due primarily to an inverted way of living, thinking, and eating.

This over-acidification leads to the over-growth in our body of micro-organisms (such as yeast and fungi) whose poisons produce the symptomologies that medical science refers to as *"disease"*.

Based on Dr. Young's theory, there's only one sickness, and there can therefore be only one remedy and treatment, and that is to **alkalize the body** and break the cycle of imbalance, thus allowing us to experience the energy, vitality and true health we're all meant to have.

What's more, Dr. Young is a man for whom I have immense respect and admiration. If you are familiar with my work (through my books, eBooks, and seminars), you know that I'm definitely not one who easily

30

buys into "miracle cures"—nor am I easily swayed by other people's opinions or anecdotal reports. I'm extremely wary of exaggerated health claims provided by individuals or enterprises that stand to make huge profits from the proliferation of those claims.

But the more I expanded my research into this New Biology™, the more I was dumbfounded by the mountains of evidence showing that this therapy has already been used by so many health practitioners who have adopted Dr Young's protocol to heal cancer and every conceivable disease.

My skepticism turned to conviction when I realized that this cure is . . .

...the only healing therapy that finally eliminates the REAL cause of cancer!

Specifically, my skepticism melted away when I saw the overwhelming evidence consisting of thousands of people that were healed of cancer and many other diseases.

This is BY FAR the simplest, most effective and most powerful therapy for curing cancer and creating optimal health. It is also the secret that both the American pharmaceutical industry and the medical establishment don't want you to know.

That's because this simple cure for virtually all diseases threatens the livelihood and the trillion-dollar earnings of the pharmaceutical and health care industries—not to mention the medical centers and physicians that make a great living from providing expensive drugs, complex medical procedures and long hospital stays.

The simple protocol which is detailed in this book represents the biggest threat to the revenues of the pharmaceutical and medical industries. It's a bigger threat than all the alternative healing therapies, nutritional supplements, natural foods and products COMBINED.

I believe it's the definitive answer to the cause, prevention and cure of cancer and of a great many diseases that plague the world today.

Therefore I am deeply honoured, thrilled and excited to introduce you to a research scientist who is not only a genius in his field, but a man with an immense heart. Dr Young is a man who truly cares deeply, and I am certain his knowledge and caring can make a difference not only in your life, but in the lives of all your family and loved ones. So let the journey of transformation begin!

31

WHAT IS CANCER?

We are very, very grateful to be able to share this research—this New Biology™—what I (Rob) refer to as a new way of living, a new way of eating, a new way of thinking.

Some of the questions we'll be covering in this chapter include:

- What is cancer?
- What's the cause of all cancer? (Is cancer a mutant cell, a virus, a mould? Or is cancer an acidic liquid?)
- Is cancer a noun or is it actually an adjective that explains what's happening to the cell?
- Are tumours bad or good?
- What role does the lymphatic system play in all this?

The focus will be on the alkaline pH of the body. The key I believe is to obtain sustainable energy.

Most of the last 25 years of my research has been focused on what is happening to the cells as it pertains specifically to the environment around those cells. And I love this quote by Ralph Waldo Emerson: "*What lies behind us and what lies before us are tiny matters compared to what lies within us.*" So the focus of my research has been on specifically what lies within us and, more specifically, how the internal fluids affect the health, energy, and vitality of the human cell. Dr Benjamin Rush, eminent physician and signer of the Declaration of Independence, said: "*Unless we put medical freedom into the Constitution, the time will come when medicine will organize into an underground dictatorship. To restrict the art of healing to one class of men and deny equal privileges to others will constitute the Bastille of medical science. All such laws are un-American and despotic.*"

As I think about my vision, the purpose of medicine I believe must include not just the treatment but also the prevention of illness and the promotion of health and fitness, rather than just focusing all of our attention on a specific diagnosis or even the treatment of disease. Because disease is an illusion, in reality disease is the body trying to prevent fermentation or break down of the tissue. It's the body in *preservation mode* trying to maintain the homeostasis of the internal fluids of the body which are *alkaline*. I believe that the ultimate purpose of medicine is to help people discover something fundamental within themselves: an awareness of the true source of wellbeing, the true source of joy, the true source of contentment that we all seek which lies in one's mind and in one's heart—which are the emotions and the spirit. This is important in order to free ourselves from the process of trying to get happiness externally, only from a physical world.

To support this approach, this theory, I believe we must begin to embrace a more spiritual vision of ourselves and of humanity as a whole, while at the right time providing great love, care, and attention to the physical body. Then, and only then, will medicine (or the treatments that medicine is currently performing) help people discover this non-physical, spiritual dimension of themselves. And when this happens I believe that we can live and work with less fear. Rather than working in fear we can work in its opposite—we can work in faith, then I believe we can truly be happy, energetic, and free.

I had the wonderful opportunity to meet with Dr Carter, who is the caretaker of the estate of Martin Luther King and also his protégé. And the most important thing that I learned about Dr Carter was his openness to not just thinking outside the box, because many of us are talking about thinking outside the box, but I would like to suggest as we contemplate these new theories that I am going to be presenting to you on the pH Miracle for cancer, that rather than thinking outside the box, we should be making the box bigger. That's right, **we don't have to think outside the box, we just need to make the box bigger** to allow new technologies, new biologies, new protocols that are effectively making the difference, specifically in the prevention and treatment of cancer.

"We must be the change we want to see."
—Ghandi

If we want to see the cure for cancer, I believe we must be the change we want to see. We'll have to look at it differently, not outside the box but inside the box making it bigger. Expanding our views and our perspective as it relates to cancer.

Now before we start exploring the pH Miracle for cancer, I must start up by saying what is a pH miracle. And I would suggest that **a pH miracle is a natural phenomenon** that is not understood currently by medical doctors, specifically **in the cause and effect relationship**. What is the cause? Is cancer a cause for disease? I say no, cancer is the body attempting to maintain homeostasis and cancer is the body in preservation mode trying to maintain the alkaline design of the human organism. So first **we must understand that cancer is unequivocally *not* a disease, but a symptom** or better yet an effect of gastrointestinal and metabolic acids that have built up in the blood and now these acids are thrown off into the tissues poisoning and suppressing our immune system making it increasingly difficult to maintain the alkaline pH of the internal fluids of the body. So these acids destroy the white cells' ability to remove acids and the cells which they spoil.

What I'm simply suggesting is that cancer is not a cell, but an acidic liquid that spoils our cells (that make up our tissues and organs) whenever acids are not properly eliminated through urination, perspiration, respiration or defecation.

Let's now look at the current medical definition of cancer: *Cancer is a group of diseases characterized by uncontrolled growth and spread of abnormal cells. If the spread is not controlled it can result in death. Cancer is caused by both external factors, some of which are known and are common in our society such as tobacco, chemicals, radiation (from our cellular phones) and internal factors: hormone imbalances, immune deficiency and gene mutations. These factors may act together in a sequence to promote what is called carcinogenesis.* This is the classical definition of cancer, taken directly from the American Cancer Society.

So what is being suggested by current medical science is that the cancer is some mutating cell (a transmutation of the genes) triggered by internal or external factors. Well this is true but what is not understood is these internal or external factors are the acids themselves. So when we're dealing with any symptom or an effect, we need to look at the cause. Whether externally or internally, the focus traditionally has been to look at the matter rather than look at the environment around the matter. And understanding the cause is very simple, just like the

34

treatment. And the New Biology™ explains the cause and effect of all sickness and disease and specifically cancer as well as how to improve the quality and quantity of life without chemical therapy, radiation or surgery.

Let me give you an example. Enervation (i.e. lack of energy), muscle weakness (you've probably seen the commercials on television) it's a new disease they call restless legs syndrome (RLS) for which there are drugs that supposedly treat the syndrome. Modern medicine wants to put everything in a disease modality—a nice little box—that has a specific treatment. Yet restless legs syndrome is weakness or loss of electrical power. It's not a disease. But by causing a flagging of the toxin elimination from the tissue, the blood becomes charged with these metabolic acids and thus the blood has to purify itself by throwing these metabolic acids into the tissues to maintain its delicate pH balance of 7.365. This is what I call the body in preservation mode, which leads to what I refer to as latent tissue acidosis. This is poison in the blood, and if that poison is not eliminated through urination, perspiration, respiration or defecation, the body has to purify itself so it throws this poison into the connective tissue. This is the disease, or is it?

Looking at the 2006 statistics for cancer in America we're looking at 1,400,000 new cases of cancer. By the way, this statistic doesn't even include skin cancer which is actually bigger than lung cancer, breast cancer or prostate cancer. And prostate cancer is known to be the leading cause of death in men while breast cancer is the leading cause of death in women. Yet when we look at cancer, the new incidents of cancer and the new diagnoses are skin cancers because skin is the third kidney—the elimination organ. And if acids are not properly eliminated through the elimination channels, then those acids accumulate beyond the toleration point, that's when a crisis takes place which means that the poison or the acid is being eliminated through the skin.

This is the reason why the blood maintains its pH by either eliminating acid through urination or throwing it into the colloidal tissue which leads to this crisis, this poisoning, this elimination through the skin, again the third kidney! And this is not a disease. The only disease is systemic, because acids flow out through your whole body. They are the waste products of metabolism. Our bodies are like cars, however

35

they're constantly on 24/7 so they require constant energy and when energy is being used, a waste product like carbon dioxide or carbon monoxide or lactic acid is being created. Acid then is constantly being created and has to be eliminated. So when energy is being used to think, to move, to breathe, at the same time an acid is being created and *acid needs to be eliminated*. If the acid is not eliminated, it is thrown out into the colloidal connective tissue. And that's our tissue that becomes the colloidal acid catcher in order to maintain the purity of the blood. The blood has to maintain the purity and this is why the blood has a constant pH. If it varies even just one point you can have ill effects. The proper balance is 7.365. If the pH starts dropping or if it starts going up, the body will do whatever it can to maintain that delicate pH. This is very significant in order to understand cancer and why it's not a cell but the spoiling of the cell and tissue by metabolic acids which are not properly eliminated because we have enervation— we don't have the energy to move the acid out to maintain the purity of the blood, so it is then sent out into the colloidal connective tissue.

When this elimination takes place through the mucus membrane of the nose for example it's called a cold—catarrh of the nose. And when these crises are repeated for years, the mucus membrane thickens and ulcerates, and the bones enlarge, closing the passages. At this stage hay fever, asthma develops. When the tonsils or any other respiratory passages become the seat of the crisis of acidity (because the acids were not properly eliminated) then we have tonsillitis, laryngitis, bronchitis, asthma, pneumonia, and cancer. You see, it's progressive, it's the same thing. All that's happening is different progressions of the same thing—just different levels of states of acidosis. When this acid is located in the cranial cavity we have dementia, Alzheimer's, Parkinson's, muddle thinking, forgetfulness. If the acids accumulate in the digestive area, we end up with irritable bowel syndrome, gastro intestinal problems, stenosis, colitis. When the acids locate in the pelvic tissue, or in the breasts, we end up with micro-calcifications as the body, in preservation mode, is using one of these alkaline buffers such as calcium to neutralize the acids and that's why we have these micro-calcifications in the pelvic area and in the breast. This always precedes the rotting of the tissue. Even in prostate cancer.

Hence all cancers are the expulsion of acids from the blood and then tissues at different points and are essentially of the same character and evolving from the one cause, namely—*systemic acidosis*—a crisis of toxaemia. The description can be extended to every organ of the body: the lung, the liver, the pancreas, the bowls, the brain, including the largest organ which has the highest incidence: the skin. Any organ that is enervated below the average standard (from stress of habit, from overstress at work, from worry, anxiety, fear, injury, etc.) may become the location of the crisis of systemic latent tissue acidosis. The symptoms show up differently depending upon which organ is being affected, which is what makes it appear as if every symptom complex is a separate and distinct disease. But we need to *not* think outside the box, we need to think inside the box, we just need to make the box *bigger*.

I give thanks to this new light shed upon nomen culture naming disease by the philosophy of The New Biology, every symptom complex goes back to the one and only cause of all so called cancers, namely *systemic latent tissue acidosis*. To find the cause of all symptomologies—lung cancer, breast cancer, brain cancer, bowl cancer, prostate cancer—we start with colds and catarrh, and watch the pathology as it travels from irritation to catarrh to inflammation to induration to ulceration and then to cancer: nothing more than rotting tissue. And what is causing the transformation (and not gene transmutation) is the spoiling of the cell due to the acids.

Have you ever opened a refrigerator and smelled the spoiling foods at the back? These are the acids! It's not some germ, it's not some virus, it's not some mold that's breaking this down, it's the acids that are breaking the tissue down and giving rise to the symptomology. **Mold is like a smoking gun, the bullet being the acid.** And yet it's not the bullet or the acid that kills, and surely not the smoke or some gene mutation, or some bacteria or virus, but it is the person himself or herself that is pulling the lifestyle and dietary trigger which then releases the acid that then tenderizes or spoils the tissue in the weakest parts of the body.

Nature's order is interfered with by innovating habits until acidosis is established. A vaccination as evidenced by the Spanish flu epidemic or an infection, in truth it's literally an out-fection from the same source causing the most vulnerable organ, specifically the bowls, to take on organic changes. The organ however has nothing to do with the cause, and directing treatment to the organ is actually compounding the problem. You cannot treat disease when in reality disease is the body in preservation trying to re-establish homeostasis in a state of systemic acidosis that's localized at the weakest part of the body.

We need to realize that breast cancer is the leading cause of death in women and that these fatty tissues (breast areas) are being used by the body to bind or collect the acids in order to protect the organs that sustain life. By the way when one does a mammogram and sees these micro-calcifications of the breast, this is an indication of a state of acidosis—the body's defensive mechanism to relieve or remove or neutralize acidity that hasn't been properly eliminated though urination, perspiration, respiration or defecation.

If we're dealing with the prostate, we're dealing with localized acidity. If we're dealing with lung cancer, we're dealing with localized acidity that can be caused by external or internal forces but everything comes from within. As we take in tobacco smoke, there are acids and toxins and poisons—one being sugar which breaks down to acetaldehyde which tenderizes this tissue. Tobacco smoking is not an addiction of nicotine, it's an addiction of sugar which causes excess acidity in a localized area. So cause is constant, ever present, always the same, only the effects change. To illustrate, a catarrh of the stomach presents first irritation, then inflammation, then ulceration and finally induration and cancer. Cancer is not what happens at first, it's the culmination of deteriorating or broken tissue spoiled by an over-acidic stomach.

Most Americans are challenged with the symptomology of indigestion which can include acid reflux, bloating, heartburn, burping, diarrhea, or even constipation. The proper way to study disease is to study health in every aspect. Disease is perverted health. Cancer is perverted health—any influence that lowers energy becomes disease producing.

There's an important question now to answer. Why do we crave sugar? It's interesting when doing an MRI or a CAT scan. What is used but radioactive sugar that is taken up by the acidic cells—not cancer cells because we don't have cancer cells, we have acidic cells or cancerous cells: cells that have been spoiled by the environment in which they live. So sugar cravings are the body's needs for sustainable energy. **Energy can only be transported through a matrix of salt.**

Therefore sugar cravings are the body's needs for salt, not sugar. And I suggest that **sugar is an acid of cellular transformation—a waste product—not a product of energy but a by-product of what the body truly uses; which is electrical potential in the form of electrons.**

The body doesn't use carbohydrates, the body uses electrons to run. The body is electrical. **Sugar is nothing more than a waste product of cellular breakdown and transformation.** Isn't that what happens to the banana? As the banana moves from irritation to inflammation to induration and then to cancer, going from green to yellow to brown, getting its "liver spots" the same way you get liver spots, through excess fermentation and rotting. We do not say the banana has cancer, we say the banana is spoiling. In the same way we shouldn't say that the lung has cancer but rather that the lung is spoiling—it is *cancerous*. **Cancer is not a noun but an adjective expressing the process of cellular transformation.** Sugar is the waste product. In fact, that's why it gets sweeter and sweeter as it ferments. In my research over the years I consistently see that we have a release of sugar from the breakdown of tissue. To overcome sugar cravings we don't have to eat sugar, we need to eat more salt. The secondary metabolites of this primary acid or sugar are acetaldehyde and ethanol alcohol. So cravings are the body's signal that the body needs more sustainable energy. We need energy to remove the acids of metabolism—the body utilizing electrons for energy purposes. Food, drinks, sun, minerals, vitamins, drugs… are common choices made by us to achieve sustainable energy, yet what we're really looking for are the *electrons* from these sources. And our choices will determine whether or not our cravings will lead to true sustainable energy which maintains the integrity of the fluids of the body and therefore the integrity of the tissues, or gives us false energy which creates this over-acidic state that leads to latent tissue acidosis which begins the process of spoiling of the tissue.

Sugar stimulates and gives the body a deceptive quick-fix—it's illusionary—whereas salt provides the matrix and gives our body the rise in sustainable energy, over a long period of time, without the high and extreme lows that come from eating an acid—whether it be sugar or any other acidic foods or drinks.

It is the skin that suffers, because if the body can't eliminate the acids that are created through energy consumption, it throws them out of the tissues and into the lymphatic system, and that's why the lymphatic system is so critical in the prevention of cancer and in the treatment of cancer, because it is the lymphatic system that is the vacuum cleaner of the acids that are in the interstitial fluids of the body, pulling these acids out in order to maintain the integrity of the tissue through diaphramic breathing and perspiration (that is if we're perspiring, which is one of the most important things we need to do on a daily basis). If we can't eliminate our acids through urination then our body urinates through the skin—which is why there is over a million cases of skin cancer a year in the United States and probably you didn't even know that. It's not talked about. Why? Because the etiology of skin cancer is not understood. It is unknown. Scientists don't know what causes basal cell carcinoma, melanoma, they do not understand it because they don't understand latent tissue acidosis and the importance of the lymphatic system as the vacuum cleaner to move the acids out via the kidneys and through perspiration. But we're not exercising, and this is why obesity and a lack of exercise have been associated with cancer—yet when we're moving our body we're moving the acids out of the tissue because the lymphatic system, unlike the circulatory system, does not have a pump (the heart), it actually flows through *movement*. It is the diaphragm muscle that acts as a pump for the lymphatic system that moves the acids through the system out through perspiration or back in the general circulation to be eliminated through urination.

If you don't want cancer, if you want to prevent it, you have to pee or eliminate your acids through urination or perspiration. And if you are a cancer sufferer you have to pee your way to health. Because cancer is not a cell, but a poisoning acidic liquid. **A cancer cell is a cell that's been spoiled or poisoned by metabolic and gastrointestinal acids. That's when the body goes into protection mode by forming fibrous materials which cross-link to encapsulate the spoiled cells and thus forming the tumour.** Hence tumour is the body's protective mechanism to encapsulate spoiled or poisoned cells from excess acids which have not been properly eliminated through urination, perspiration, defecation, and respiration. The tumour is the body's solution to protect healthy cells and tissues. So the tumour is not the problem. Let the tumour go. Let it do its job. The focus must be placed not on the tumour but on the *environment* around the tumour which is full of acids, and one of the common acids which is in higher concentration around all tumours is lactic acid, because **lactic acid is a by-product of sugar metabolism when we're in a state of oxygen deprivation**. **So cancer is a *systemic acidic condition* that settles in the weakest parts of the body, not a local problem that metastasizes.** You see metastasis is localized acids that spoil other cells much like a rotten apple spoiling the bushel of other healthy apples.

There is no such thing as a cancer cell. A cancer cell is in reality a *cancerous* cell, it's an *adjective* expressing the spoiling cell that's spoiling in an over-acidic environment. A cancerous cell was once a healthy cell that has been spoiled from an over-acidic lifestyle and diet and the body's inability to move these acids through the proper channels of elimination. **The only solution** then to the acidic liquids that poison our body cells causing the effect that medical doctors call cancer, **is to change the environment**. It has to be a contextual approach. *We must maintain the alkaline design of the human body.* **This has been the great discovery of the 21st century—that the human organism is alkaline by design** (every part that makes up every anatomical element that makes up our genetic material that makes up our cells, every single part has to be bathed in an alkaline fluid which needs to be changed every 48 hours).

Early in the 19th century, beginning on January 17, 1912, a famous French physiologist of the Rockefeller Institute and Nobel Prize winner, Dr. Alexis Carrel, removed a very small piece of heart muscle from an unhatched chicken embryo—still warm and living—and placed it in fresh nutrient solution in a glass flask of his design. He transferred the tissue every forty-eight hours, during which time it doubled in size and had to be trimmed before being moved to its new flask. And every time he moved it he would put it into an alkaline saline solution with the appropriate alkalizing minerals. Thirty years later the tissue was still growing. Keep in mind that the average chicken lives for 5-7 years. So after getting bored of singing "Happy Birthday" to the chicken heart for over thirty years he decided to pull the plug and not change the fluids every 48 hours and the heart died.

This is a very important discovery (which very few people know about) because it answers the question about why cells live. You see, the life expectancy of the human cell is infinite. It just becomes compromised. Once we understand that matter cannot be created nor can it be destroyed it can only change its form or function, then we realize that the environment is everything, the terrain is everything, and the cell is subservient to that. The secret to Dr. Carrel's chicken heart surviving for thirty years lies in this knowledge, this new biology, this new way of living and thinking as we expand the box not think outside the box, that the cell is only as healthy as the fluids it is bathed in. The heart is only as healthy as the cells. If you have lung cancer, that is an expression of the environment. And the cell as it's breaking down is the smoke of the gun.

Carrel's experiment brought us to the modern new biology, the new understanding, the new expansion, and the new definition of cancer— that the composition of our body fluids that bathe the outside of our cells must be controlled very carefully from moment to moment and day to day with no single important constituent varying more than a few percent. This can be controlled and you can do it yourself!

In 1932 Otto Warburg received his Nobel Prize in medicine for discovering the cause of cancer. He described it as a cell changing its mode of respiration, its mode of metabolism—from respiration to fermentation. He suggested that cancer was the result of an acidic environment, a state of oxygen deprivation. He showed that cancer thrives in anaerobic (without oxygen), or acidic, conditions. In other words, the main cause for cancer is acidity of the human body.

Most doctors and multi billion dollar drug companies, for instance, are focused on the wrong causes of disease. Some claim that *viruses, microbes, germs* or *harmful bacteria* are the cause of cancer. Others say it's the *toxins* in the food we eat, the air we breathe and the substances we consume. And still others blame our *genes* or *stress* or *aging* or *hormonal imbalance* for the common health issues that beset most people.

While all of these factors may *characterize* most diseases, or might be *precursors* or *by-products* of disease, they do not CAUSE disease. Rather, **they bring about a condition in the body that, in turn, causes disease**. Whether you call it over-acidity, over-acidification, acid-overload, or acidosis, it boils down to too much acid waste in your body.

Warburg also wrote a paper entitled, "The Prime Cause and Prevention of Cancer." He states: "There is no disease whose prime cause is better known. Over acidity."

In 1966 Warburg finished one of his most famous speeches with the following statement: **"Nobody today can say that one does not know what the prime cause of cancer is. On the contrary, there is no disease whose prime cause is better known, so that today ignorance is no longer an excuse for avoiding measures for prevention."** [The Prime Cause and Prevention of Cancer. Dr. Otto Warburg Lecture delivered to Nobel Laureates on June 30, 1966 at Lindau, Lake Constance, Germany]

When we understand this we realize that all conditions of cancer can potentially be reversed if the treatments are focused on the fluids not the cell. Therefore it doesn't matter what the cancer is, because **cancer is not the cause but the effect of an over-acidic lifestyle and diet which *is* the cause**. It's the person pulling the lifestyle and dietary trigger.

After 25 years of doing blood research, after looking at thousands and thousands of cancer patients, I've never seen healthy blood or an alkaline environment—whether testing the pH of the saliva, or the urine, or the blood, or the sweat, or the tears—they are all acidic in an over-acidic environment. And after 25 years I've learned that the human organism is alkaline by design and acidic by function, and if we but maintain this alkaline design of our body through an alkaline lifestyle and diet we will prevent all cancers. For the cure of cancer is not found in its treatment, because again cancer or a cancerous condition is the body in preservation mode trying to maintain alkalinity, so the cure is going to be found not in its treatment of the tissue but in maintaining the alkaline design of the human fluids of the body. As Thomas Edison said: "The doctor of the future will give no medicine, but will involve the patient in the proper use of food, fresh air and exercise."

THE PH MIRACLE FOR CANCER

The cure, the prevention, the reversal for cancer is not found in the treatment of tissue, but rather in maintaining the alkaline design of the human organism, and the most important test that you can do to determine whether you are in a state of over-acidity is testing the pH of the fluids.

So are tumors bad or good? They are good because they are the expression of the body in preservation mode trying to prevent healthy tissue from spoiling. What role does the lymphatic system play in cancer? A critical role to move acids out of the interstitial fluids of the body and to move those through the pores of our skin or back into circulation to be eliminated through urination.

What is the cause of prostate cancer? It is a systemic problem that localizes at the weakest part, i.e. prostate, which is the first cause of death in men, prostate cancer. It's the number one cause, and the number two cause of death in women is breast cancer. Do you realize that 50% of the men on the planet will sometime in their life have the incidence or the expression of over-acidity that's going to be called cancer. The risk factors for women are one in three. You see, once we understand that cancer is not a cell but a liquid that spoils cells, and we begin the process of maintaining this alkaline design—*this understanding by the way is very empowering!*—then with this knowledge and conviction we can make a commitment to change. And I'm so grateful to be able to share this knowledge with you of the new biology, and this one sickness, this one disease, this one cause for cancer, the systemic poisoning of the tissues as the blood tries to maintain its delicate pH because the body is either congested or does not have the energy to move these acids, these poisonous, toxic fluids out through urination or perspiration. It is the only cause.

Cancer Is A Four Letter Word: ACID

The physical aspects have to be considered before we can bring our emotional state back into balance, and of course there is a bowel-blood-brain connection and so the mental body can be disconnected if our physical body—particularly the bowels—are not balanced in terms of maintaining health and energy and alkalinity in the bowels. This is what I call the pyramid of life or the teeter-totter of life and the key here is to maintain homeostasis not only biochemically between acid and alkaline, but also bioenergetically between protons and electrons.

So we're going to be focusing on an alkalizing lifestyle. We're going to be focusing on an alkalizing diet. We're going to be focusing on lifestyles and diets that are electron rich so they're contributing energy to our lives since our bodies run on energy and electricity rather than on the acidic aspects or the proton concentrations which are found in many of our food stuffs, in our nutritional supplements, and in many lifestyle choices that can affect this teeter-totter.

According to the pH Miracle science, on a scale from 0-10, cancer is a state of over acidity at the highest level—a natural phenomenon that is currently not understood by current medical savants. There is not a well understood definition other than what the American Cancer Society has actually written in their reports that cancer is a mutation of the cell. Well we need to roll this back—what is causing the mutation of the cell? That mutation is being caused by liquids or acids that are disturbing or breaking down the human cell or the animal cell or the plant cell.

So again the questions are: What is cancer, what is the cause of all cancer, is cancer a mutant cell or a virus or a mold or an acidic liquid, what causes the #1 cancer in women (that's breast cancer), what causes the #1 cancer in men (this is prostate cancer), is cancer a noun, a verb, an adjective; is cancer something we catch or something we do, are tumors good or bad, what role does the lymphatic system play in cancer?

Basically, cancer is a liquid, it's an acidic liquid, created from energy consumption. So it's a waste product of metabolism and cellular breakdown. What is the cause of all cancers? The cause is an over acidic state brought on primarily by lifestyle and dietary choices. Is cancer a mutant cell? No, it's a fermenting cell that's broken down by acidic toxic waste. So what causes the #1 cancer in women? Acid. Acid being thrown into breast cancer—we're going to cover that in a minute. Prostate cancer—the same thing. Cancer is not a noun. It's actually a description of what's happening to the cells. So it's an adjective. We don't have a cancer cell, we have a *cancerous* cell. Is cancer something we catch? No it's not something we catch, it's something that WE DO through our lifestyle and it's an EFFECT of the cause and effect relationship. Are tumors good or bad? I would suggest to you that tumors are the body's way of encapsulating these morbid cells that have been spoiled by acids that are not properly eliminated through urination or perspiration, and that all tumors are nothing more than fibrin that is being created cross-linked to encapsulate these morbid cells in order to maintain the integrity of the healthy cells. Much like a rotten apple will spoil all of the healthy apples in a bushel of apples, we need to encapsulate that apple or encapsulate those cells in order to preserve the health of all the other healthy cells, or they'll spoil too as well. That gives rise to the lymphatic system and its important role.

The role of the lymphatic system is to *move acid out of the tissues* so it doesn't spoil your cells. That's why there are so many lymphatic cancers, because once the lymphatic system pulls the acid out of the tissue if it doesn't move it out through perspiration because you're not exercising, or it doesn't move it back into circulation and you don't urinate it, then the lymphatic system becomes congested and this is the reason for Hodgkin's and non-Hodgkin's lymphomas and the reasons why lymph nodes become enlarged and inflamed is because they're full of these acidic toxins that are not being properly eliminated through perspiration or back through circulation through urination.

So the new questions then are where does cancer begin, does diet & lifestyle have anything to do with cancer, is cancer preventable and if so how do we prevent it, and if I have cancer such as lung, colon, prostate, breast, or pancreatic cancer can I reverse it without having traditional chemical therapy, radiation, or even surgery?

According to the American Cancer Society Cancer Facts and Figures 2006, new cancer cases this year: 1,399,000. Males: 720,000. Females: 679,000. Estimated deaths this year in the United States: 564,830. New breast cancer cases: 212,000; that's 31% of all cancers! Estimated deaths this year: up to 41,000. And the interesting thing Denmark is #1 in breast cancers at 27% where the U.S. is at 19%. So this is an epidemic worldwide and I want women to understand what's causing this because women are at 100% risk for breast cancer. Estimated deaths for prostate cancer is 27,800 and 79% in the U.S.; Uganda #1 for prostate cancer at 32%, U.S. at 28% and new cases for prostate cancer 234,000. I mean here again this is also an epidemic—greater than lung cancers.

In 2008, there were 1,437,199 new cancer cases in the US. It is estimated that 2,220,692 new cases of cancer will occur in the US in the year 2030—a 55 percent increase! (Mexico will experience a 52 percent increase by 2030, Canada will experience a 66 percent increase.) These statistics are staggering!

One of the reports that came out by Food, Nutrition and Prevention of Cancer: A Global Perspective (a 700 page report) actually shows the foods that will prevent cancer. You'll notice here at the bottom that vegetables in all categories will actually prevent cancers, and fruits too, but vegetables are the strongest particularly in lung and stomach and pancreatic cancer and colorectal cancer and breast cancer, even bladder cancers, but what is killing us, as we look at the study—and this was a 10 year study, a worldwide study that was funded by the World Health Organization—alcohol and smoking. Alcohol causes liver cancer—we all know that—and if we look at lung cancer it increases threefold if we, of course, smoke too as well. Alcohol and smoking are the two major dietary and lifestyle *choices*—that we make!—that cause the majority of cancers. Even breast cancer is showing this particularly in women. So alcohol is one of the major contributors to breast cancer and if you'll also notice it's also associated with obesity and in the book *The pH Miracle for Weight Loss* I've already shared with the world that obesity is the body's way of protecting itself against excessive acidity. So we pack on the pounds to park our acids that aren't being eliminated through urination or perspiration or respiration or defecation. So obesity is definitely a factor. So I wanted to share some of these statistics with you as we look at this.

Now going back to the question what is cancer, what is the origin of cancer, where does it start? Very simply I want to tell you *it starts in our choices*. Before we put anything into our mouth it starts with choice. We choose to smoke or not. We choose to drink alcohol or not. These are choices we make. We can choose not to drink alcohol. We can choose not to smoke and we're going to reduce our risk but it starts with *choice*. It's not some phantom virus or some mutant cell, it's choice that causes cancer. And in our acidic lifestyle and dietary choices, cancer—and this is a very important discovery—cancer is not a cell, but a poisonous, acidic liquid that's poisoned cells. So a cancer cell is a cell that has been spoiled or poisoned by metabolic or gastrointestinal acids. A tumor, therefore, is when a group of cells have been spoiled, that's when a tumor forms. Just like a scab is formed. A scab is made up of the same material a tumor is made up of. It's the body protective mechanism to encapsulate spoiled or poisoned cells from excess acids that have not been properly eliminated through urination, perspiration, defecation, or respiration. The tumor is like the scab that forms itself when you cut your finger. It's the body's solution to protect healthy cells and tissues. So cancer is a systemic acidic condition—in liquid form—that flows through every part of our body and settles at the weakest parts of the body. Somebody says, "Well why does it settle in the breasts?" Well it settles in the breasts because that's a fatty tissue and that's the way the body protects itself by throwing acid out into the breast tissue or out into the brain tissue or out into the fatty tissue in the buttocks or thighs to protect the organs that sustain life.

So cancer is a systemic acidic condition that settles in the weakest part of the body rather than a localized problem that metastasized; where a metastasis is nothing more than a localized acidity that spoils other cells much like a rotten apple spoiling a bushel of healthy apples. It's a domino effect. It's not a creation of a new cell that's improperly being created. There's no such thing as a cancer cell. This is the scientific illusion. This is what we've been told to believe. In reality a cancer cell was once a healthy animal, plant, human cell that's been spoiled from its waste products. To move, to breathe, to think the body produces waste products; if these toxins are not eliminated they have to be put somewhere and so they're thrown out into the fatty tissues. That's why all women are at risk for breast cancer. The tumor then is not the problem but the solution to protect healthy cells and tissues from being spoiled from other rotting cells and tissues. The only solution to the acidic liquids that poison body cells causing the effect is to alkalize and energize the body. This is what we teach in all of our books.

So we must understand that the human body is alkaline by design and acidic by function—breathing, thinking, moving is acidic, but our body is designed to move those acids out properly if we're eating the right kinds of foods and do not become over acidic. Therefore if we want a healthy body we must maintain that alkaline design. As an example I often use, that's what happens to healthy grapefruits that turn to cancer: they don't get old, they mold, and this is what happens to us. We ferment. Again, much like a banana that goes from green to yellow to brown, it actually is fermenting, and mold and bacteria and yeast are just the evidence that the tissue is breaking down; spoiled by acidity. It even comes out through the skin. If you've got skin problems this is what it looks like when acids have actually disturbed the cells as the cells begin to transform and move these acids out through the third kidney: the skin. And so as we look at the different stages of acidity that's causing damage to the epithelial cells, we see stage 0 to stage I to stage II to stage III to stage IV as this acidity is not contained and so it's disturbing more cells and it looks as if it's metastasizing, or the tumor is growing, but in reality it's actually encapsulating even more tissue that's being spoiled from the fact that what has not changed is our personal lifestyle and dietary choices. If we want to reverse stage IV, stage III, stage II, stage I cancer we have to do it with lifestyle and dietary choices.

Otto Warburg said this in his 1966 lecture, I quote, "The prime cause of cancer is in the replacement of respiration of oxygen in normal body cells by fermentation of sugar. All normal body cells meet their energy needs by respiration of oxygen, whereas cancer cells meet their energy needs in great part by fermentation. All normal body cells are thus obligate aerobes whereas all cancer cells are partial anaerobes. From the standpoint of the physics and chemistry of life, this difference between normal and cancer cells is so great that one can scarcely picture a greater difference. Oxygen gas, the donor of energy in plants and animals, is dethroned in the cancer cells, or the cancerous cells, and replaced by an energy yielding reaction of the lowest living forms, namely fermentation of glucose." I would somewhat qualify that in that as the cells are using electrical energy the glucose is actually the acid that's being eliminated and that's because we do not run our bodies on sugar, we run our bodies on *electrons*, and sugar is the acidic waste product of cellular breakdown and this is the reason why blood sugars increase in type 1 diabetics. Well Otto Warburg received the Nobel Prize in 1932 when he discovered that when the pH is off oxygen falls, cells then change from an aerobic state to an anaerobic environment giving rise to fermentation or increased acidity and of course cancer is nothing more than the result of an acidic environment. Once we realize that then we can make better lifestyle and dietary choices.

THE TRUE CAUSE OF CANCER

As a point of review, the alkaline pH of the body is paramount. It is literally the key to sustain our energies, and I think what we're really seeking for is not just having energy during the day, but sustainable energy, energy that's not going up and down and up and down where we're trying to somehow fake our body into moving rather than having enough reserves to be able to draw on those particular energy reserves so that our body can be sustained for longer durations or longer periods of time. That's what I believe is significant because the body runs on electricity, electrical potential. We eat food for electrical potential, and when we don't have the energy, we lack energy, which is a word called enervation, and when we go to enervation, we actually block elimination. So we move from energy to enervation to elimination; when elimination is actually blocked, then we start absorbing our own waste products and that's something we want to avoid at all costs. And so in order to tell what impact that acidity is having on our system, we measure the pH; which is probably the most important measurement that we should be measuring on a daily basis in order to maintain our health energy and vitality.

So as we talk about this pH miracle—a natural phenomenon that's not understood by current medical savants—it's critically important that we just ingrain this into our consciousness: this **cause and effect relationship**.

To find the cause of any symptom... for example recently I received a call from a husband whose spouse (47 years old, non smoker) had lung cancer. Small cell carcinoma—and they sent her home to die. Her death train is running faster than her life train, and they've got her hooked up to an IV of sugar, as if sugar is going to somehow keep the energy that she needs. Well she can't move. She can't even speak anymore now. Her eliminations have been checked and she's on a catheter and she has no control of her bowels. This all starts with the body going into preservation mode when it starts building up catarrh or bound up acids with sodium bicarbonate, and if you watch the pathology, it travels from irritation to catarrh, inflammation, induration, ulceration and then to degeneration or what we call cancer. And to try to find the cause of any particular symptom, even if we look at all the statistics, the cancer figures and facts—prostate cancer, breast cancer—the number one cause of death in women is breast cancer. The number one cause of death in men is prostate cancer. What is the cause of prostate cancer? What is the cause of breast cancer?

Nature's order is interfered with by enervation and enervating habits. Those are habits that are pulling energy from the body until acidosis is established. Systemic acidosis that mobilizes to the weakest part of the body. Take a vaccination, as evidenced in the Gulf War Syndrome or even the Spanish flue epidemic or any type of so-called infection that seems to happen during the holiday seasons when we're overindulging in high acidic foods, you know alcohol, pastries, meats, dairies. These are all high acidic foods. And they act as a fire brand in causing the most vulnerable organ, which is the bowels, to take on organic change. This organ however has nothing to do with the cause, and directing treatment to this organ is compounding the problem. Types of such nonsense are even blood transfusions for pernicious anemia; gland treatment for gland impotency; cutting out stones or ulcers or tumors; and the latest craziness is preventative breast cancer by doing a voluntary mastectomy.

There's no question that one of the most pernicious practices in vogue today is treating so called disease with disease. Now I want you to think about treating disease with disease. That is immunizing with products of disease. Current medical science calls this pathological thinking *vaccination* and it even includes the treatments that are chemically acidic-based related, particularly in cancer, such as chemical therapy. If cause is not known, how is prevention or cure possible? As for example, by producing a mild form of small pox vaccine or other so called disease by poisoning a healthy person by introducing into the body the pathological products of that said disease? Certainly only pathological thinking can arrive at such conclusions. Metabolic acids are made from the products of disease, and the idea that disease can be induced (by vaccines or chemical therapy) to cure itself is a product of pathological thinking.

> *"The only safe vaccine is one that is never used."*
> Dr. James R. Shannon, former Director,
> National Institute of Health

Now listen closely: if prevention and cure mean producing disease, surely prevention and cure are not desirable. If prevention can't be accomplished, then cures will not be needed. It is not disease, it is cause in all of its aspects that we need to know before we can take steps to prevent or cure disease.

So as we look at our earlier questions, what is cancer? What is the cause of all cancers? What is the cause of the #1 cancer: breast cancer for women, prostate cancer for men? Is cancer a noun or a verb? Is cancer something we catch or something we do? Are tumors good or bad? What role does the lymphatic system play? Where does cancer begin? Does diet and lifestyle have anything to do with cancer? Is cancer preventable? If I have cancer, such as lung, colon, prostate or breast, what about having chemical therapy? Think about it. Radiation… do we use disease approaches in treating disease?

The phenomenon that takes place in an over acidic body is the documentation of biological transformation and how healthy cells become cancerous cells. This is actually published and documented (March 15, 1967), and this paper appeared in the Annals of the New York Academy of Sciences, volume 141. A lot of folks don't realize that pleomorphism is not something that's made up — biological transformation is real. It was documented over a hundred years ago by Antoine Bechamp when he documented a body cell transforming into bacteria, Royal Rife saw the same thing, Dr. Livingston Wheeler saw the same thing. It was documented by over a hundred scientists in a published paper in the Annals of the New York Academy of Sciences where they actually documented long filamentous forms appearing when cultured on von Brehmer's medium. Due to its remarkable pleomorphism, the organism was capable of resembling micrococci, diphtheroids, bacilli, fungi, viruses, and host cell inclusions. So from an elongated cell—like a bacterial rod—it transformed into a coccus—or a round bacterial form—with a clear tendency towards aggregation, this is by the way what they call streptococcus. I know everybody freaks out about bacteria. We've been talking in the papers about E. coli, we're talking about staph and strep and these types of infections, which in reality are out-fections. When I say out-fections, they're coming from the cells as they transform.

What most folks don't realize is what's happening in an oxygen deprived environment, that the anatomical living elements that make up any matter are transforming the matter. So we don't have species-specific bacteria or species-specific yeast or species-specific molds. The molds in yeast and bacteria are transformations of what used to be healthy matter of cells that are transforming to adapt to an oxygen deprived environment. And this was documented over a hundred years ago by Bechamp and it was documented by our own scientists and published in the Annals of New York Academy of Sciences in '67, and then it was documented again, unbeknownst to me.

I had no idea. I thought I was looking at something for the first time when I actually documented an anthrax-like bacteria, that had appendages attached to it, literally transform. What I was actually witnessing was a biological transformation (as seen on pg. 126 of my book "Sick and Tired") of a bacterial rod (bacillus) transforming into a spherical form (coccus) very much the same dimensions of a red blood cell. Then you'll see two bulges on the surface of the membranes actually pushing out which is the birth of two platelets. I knew for the first time that bacteria was not a demon, not an entity but a transformation, a new formation of a preceding form. Not the cause of disease but the expression of a change in the internal environment which had given rise to change. Bacteria can then be understood not so much as the cause of disease, but as a result of an imbalanced, overly acidic milieu. A simple example is a packaged loaf of bread beyond its expiration date that is growing mold. It is not an outside invader that has ruined the bread, but an unsuitable environment.

And by the way what comes out of this bacterial rod is, as you can also watch it on YouTube: http://youtu.be/gQnWvaQCr-w, is a Y single membrane yeast cell: Y form yeast is coming right out of the bacterial cell and in turn gives birth to two platelets. That's why I came up with this conclusion that platelets were nothing more than filthy, dirty, little bacterial cells, and for a microbiologist to say that openly to a group of doctors or other microbiologists… they call that "heresy" and want to put me to the stake for saying platelets are actually bacterial cells that are born out of cellular degeneration but this is what's happening. Cells are transforming. They're not species-specific. And yet we're in the business of categorizing everything, and so we treat E. coli as if it's some sort of species or some form that's invading our bodies which is literally not true. It's a transformation of matter as it's transforming based upon its environment.

54

So when we get to the cause… Cause is constant, ever present and always the same. Only the effects and the object on which cause acts change and the changes are most inconstant. To illustrate, a catarrh of the stomach (and catarrh is just bound up acids with basically elemental buffers like sodium bicarbonate) presents first irritation, then inflammation, then ulceration and finally induration and cancer. It's a progressive change of the cells as the environment is changing. And not all cases run true to form; only a small percentage evolve to ulcerations, and a few reach the cancer stage. More exit by way of acute food poisoning or acute indigestion than by chronic diseases. Most Americans are challenged with the symptomology of indigestion, which can include acid reflux which is very popular these days, bloating, that's also very popular, indigestion, diarrhea and also constipation.

The proper way to study disease—to study cancer—is to study health in every aspect—*every aspect*. Disease is perverted health. There's nothing special about it. Cancer is just perverted health. Any influence that lowers our energy becomes disease. Disease cannot be its own cure. That's why you don't use chemotherapy. Neither can it be its own prevention. My discovery of the truth that all cancers, all sickness and disease—and acid being the cause of all so called diseases—came about slowly, it didn't happen just all at once. So as we're looking at all these questions, these answers have come after 25 years of not just research (that is, research and reading) but actually seeing the effects of what's happening to clients, patients that are changing their internal environment and seeing those changes at the cellular level.

Here are some new questions: What impact do our emotions have on our health? What influences do our emotions have on causing, reversing or preventing cancer? How do our thoughts impact the success of the treatment for cancer? Can you cause cancer with your thoughts? And how does your personal relationship with your friends, your family, your spouse either prevent or can it cause cancer?

Earlier I showed you the teeter-totter of life, and the foundation of that teeter-totter—my four food groups—water, salt, chlorophyll and fats. We have to start out with the physiology because the next tier on our pyramid is the emotional body-energy in motion. Emotion is energy in motion—that affects our mental body and all of this combined affects our spiritual body, which creates what we call the soul. The soul is a heterogeneous solution of two or more dissimilar ingredients that are bound up into one. So we have the physical body, the emotional body, the mental body and the spiritual body which creates the soul of the body, or the soul of man.

And in order to get the body back into a state of homeostasis—or balance—you have to start with the physiology, and you have to start with balancing the acid/alkaline balance. That's why it's so important to measure the pH of the fluids of the body. They have to be at least 7.2 or better.

As we think about the cause or the consequence, we have to think about the choice. So it begins with sensitivity and it leads up gradually, as we become more acidic, to degeneration. These are just different stages of levels of acidosis. There's nothing in the name; there's nothing that we gain or learn from calling a disease cancer or calling a disease MS. That doesn't tell us anything. It tells us though, once we understand the new biology, that this person is highly acidic; that they're absorbing their own waste products; that their choice of lifestyle and diet is affecting them. It's just not what you eat, it's also what you think. It's how you live. It's your thoughts. Your thoughts are part of your lifestyle and what you eat impacts the internal fluids of the body, which impacts the health of the tissue; that leads either to health, energy and vitality or to a state of latent tissue acidosis or crisis of toxemia.

So there's a law of the universe. The law of the universe is called the duality of life, and the duality of life suggests there needs to be opposition in all things that we might learn by experience. How do we understand something if we do not have choice? We have to have choice. In the duality of life, especially within our emotions, we can either go to the emotion of fear or we can go to the emotion of faith. This is duality. We can live in the past. We can fear the future—which is basically a fear-based emotion from my perspective—or we can live in faith. One who lives in faith is one, I believe, who is focused on what is happening now. They're not necessarily concerned about the past because the past is over. They're concerned about what is happening now and how am I controlling this duality of life, this law of the universe. And so the acronym for fear is False Evidence

Appearing Real because most of what we think about generally never happens. When we actually move from fear to faith, and of course I've come up with an acronym for faith: First Attribute In Thinking Healthy. That's what I believe faith is. It's healthy thinking and it's the first attribute of conviction that one has to have in order to begin controlling the consequences that roll back to the choices that we're making, which is *choice equals consequence*. So if we are unhealthy, then we've made unhealthy choices.

So where does cancer begin? It begins with our choice. And if we're experiencing good health, we have made good choices. And if we're experiencing ill health, we have made poor choices. I believe that we need to understand this law of the universe because without this law there would be no choice—there'd be nothing to choose from. You either choose evil or you choose good. You choose acidic foods or you choose alkaline foods. Without that choice there can be no consequences. We then experience the consequences of our choice in this duality of life, and we can either live in a state of fear or we can live, I believe, in a state of faith. I believe that if you move to a state of faith that many of the consequences you experience will change significantly.

For example, this is an estimation based upon the pH scale. The pH scale is exponential. For every point it moves, it moves to the power of 10. So if I have a scale from 1 to 14 and 7 is the mid point, if our body fluids are slightly alkaline at 7.2, if my body fluids or any fluid for that matter moved from 7 to 8, that would be a 10 times increase. And for each time it moves, it goes from 7 to 8 ten times, 8 to 9 is 100 times; 9-10 is 1,000 times. I would like to suggest to you that negative thoughts and feelings initially and long-term can lower the pH of the urine by 1,000 times.

Now I can prove this quite simply... If you want to catch yourself you test your pH. If you've been testing your pH over a period of time on a daily basis, and for some reason something has truly upset you—for a good reason or for no good reason for that matter—test your pH after that emotion, and you'll notice that your pH has decreased significantly anywhere from 10 to 1,000 times. This can cause the body to go into preservation mode 24/7 using up its alkaline buffering reserves. If the body is using its alkalinity and its energy to neutralize

57

the acidity off an emotion, emotions are most definitely contributing to a state of acidity or alkalinity which also then equates to a state of health, energy or wellness or a state of sickness and disease. Because once the alkaline reserves are used up by the body, the body goes into body wasting. It starts wasting the bone, it starts wasting the muscle to pull alkaline buffers to neutralize the acidity in the blood in order to maintain alkalinity.

And finally, if you stay within those emotions, you die a miserable person. You do not change to be a happy person upon death. Death is not the solution; life is the solution. Life problems can either make you a better person or a bitter person. And you can test this chemistry. You can measure it. You can measure the pH of the saliva. You can measure the pH of the urine. And you can see the biological changes, the biochemical changes that take place as the pH lowers when you're in a state of emotional stress. Over a period of time this can rage havoc to the tissues because if the body becomes enervated—and enervation leads to congested eliminations—then you start absorbing your own urine. When you start absorbing your own waste products, you start tenderizing your bones, your heart, your brain, your breasts, your prostate, and this is what causes them to physiologically break down. So our thoughts and feelings do impact our physiology. Our physiology affects our emotions, and our emotions affect our physical body. This, I believe, is a fact and it can be measured biochemically.

So are you having a thought attack? I would suggest that most heart attacks or cancers are brought on by our thoughts. Thoughts require energy. Are we using our energy to move our bodies in a positive way? Or are we using energy to move our bodies in a negative way? When we use energy and when energy's consumed, guess what is the byproduct of that? It's an acid and if you don't have the energy to move that acid out, it goes into the breast tissue, the brain tissue, the prostate; it's thrown out into the organs, away from the organs that sustain life. It begins very simply with just sensitivities. Like I said catarrh, irritation, inflammation, aches and pains—these are the body's signals. Relating this to a car, is our body honking or is our body humming? If it's honking, we're feeling the honking signals—the irritation, the inflammation, the sensitivities. You see aches and pains lead to cancerous tissues, and they all can begin with our thoughts.

58

So while we're in these negative thoughts, all of a sudden you start thinking, "Wow, I need more energy." And so what happens? You look for sugar. We've been taught that sugar is a source of energy and we become addicted to this drug. Most people don't realize that sugar is an acid from cellular breakdown. It's not a compound for energy. It's actually a *waste product* of cellular degeneration. Our sugar cravings are the body crying out for sustainable energy. Energy can only be transferred through a matrix of salt. Therefore, sugar cravings are the need for salt—not sugar—and for foods that actually release electrical potential to energize the anatomical elements that make up our cells in our bodies. When we move to sugar, we poison ourselves and do not provide the matrix to which energy can be then transferred.

Sugar then is the primary metabolite of fermentation. By ferments—ferments are the anatomical elements that make up our genetic matter and are not a source of energy—all we're doing is poisoning ourselves. These sugars can break down to other metabolites, one being vinegar. It's a secondary metabolite. It's called acetaldehyde and the third one is called ethanol alcohol. These are serious neurotoxins which lead to brain cancer. So I want you to remember this—because you're probably hearing this for the first time—sugar is a waste product. It's a ferment from cellular transformation. It's *not* a fuel for energy. Our bodies do *not* run on sugar. Our bodies run on electricity and that electricity is transported through a matrix of salt, and when you crave something and you literally go to the sugar, you're doing that from your thought processes because of what you've identified from your past experiences—what you learned and what you're taught at home or at school—that sugar is a source of energy and we become addicted to that.

The last thing that we should be going to, as most people don't know that, is that cancer cells uptake the sugar. They live within their own waste products. They literally float within their own urine. So when you're getting an MRI, your body's infused with radioactive sugar and that radioactive sugar is literally taken up by the cancerous cells. Not the cancer cell—because there's no such thing—but the *cancerous* cells. So cravings of sugar are the body's signal that it needs more sustainable energy; food, drink, sun, minerals, vitamins and drugs are the common choices made by us to achieve sustainable energy. Our choices will determine, between this duality of life, the consequence of

59

whether we're healthy or sick, and whether or not our cravings will lead to true sustainable energy or false energy. You don't get energy from drinking coffee. All you prove is you can poison yourself and the body going into preservation mode to release stored energy. Sugar will stimulate and give the body a quick fix of energy whereas salt will give the body the gradual rise in energy to sustain over a longer period of time without the high and the extreme low that comes from eating sugar or other acidic foods.

As a society, since we don't understand these foundational principles, we come up with these ridiculous ideas that in order to prevent cancer, we need to remove our breasts as if we have some familiar genetic predisposition to breast cancer, so let's take the breasts off to prevent that. Well, how many men would take off their testicles to prevent testicle cancer? I wouldn't see a bunch of men lining up for that. This is madness. Your body craves salt not sugar. It is the matrix of energy distribution. Salt is the element that makes all thought possible. You can't even have an emotion without salt. It makes movement possible. It makes your heart beat. Salt is the foundation for hydration and alkalinity of the extracellular fluids. Salt is the element that provides the matrix through which the endocrine glands communicate. Often they say, "Well this cancer is hormone dependent," as if it has something to do with testosterone. Testosterone and estrogen are the waste products of those glands using energy. You don't need hormones; you need salt. It's the quickest fix to balancing the endocrine system. Without salt, there's no thought. There's no emotion. There's no energy in motion. There's no energy; there's no sustainable energy; there's no organized life. This is why our blood is salted with sodium chloride not sugar. Salt is simply the savior of our physical bodies and it helps to maintain that alkaline balance which helps to maintain that peaceful feeling that comes not only in our physical body, but in our emotional and mental and spiritual body as we provide the foundational alkalinity.

The purpose of the endocrine system is to support the energy demands of the body during a flight or fight response, to support the alkaline design of the human organism to help mediate the fluids of acidosis out through elimination. The endocrine system is our wireless system that sends informational signals to varying parts of the body via a matrix of salt. Hormones—and I know many of you are hearing this for the first time—are the poisonous acidic waste products of the

60

endocrine glands when consuming energy during glandular communication. No one needs more acidic hormones. We balance the hormones when we provide the foundational elemental energy in those foods that carry electrical energy, those fluids that carry electrical potential. Health is energy and energy is health, and the endocrine system is the body's delivery system which helps to manage that energy system when it's out of whack, and we see this a lot in our society because we're all moving to choices that create the consequences of an over acidic body from an over acidic lifestyle and diet. So we end up with blood that looks like this:

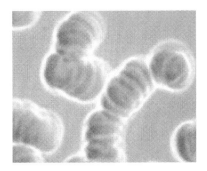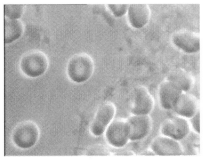

It's all stacked. It can't circulate properly. There's more yeast. They say, "Well this is from a yeast infection." There's no such thing as a yeast infection. Yeast is born within us, not from without us. When we see yeast in the blood, this is not some sort of invasion, no more than there is an invasion from some other phantom virus. It doesn't come from the outside, it comes from the inside. Through documented, scientific verification that pleomorphism is a reality; that yeast is a transformation much like a caterpillar morphing into a butterfly, it's one of the culminant forms of biological transformation as the pH begins to drop and our fluids become more acidic. This has to be monitored on a regular basis, but what doctor in the country or literally in the world is doing this on a regular basis? We're not looking at the pH. We're not looking at the state or the congestion or the quality of the fluids of our bodies and the quality of the cells. We're not measuring the liters of yeast in the bloodstream, and yet they're always present in a condition of imbalance.

So when we look at the coagulated blood, we see the blood is over acidic, we see that it cannot coagulate properly, and that's brought on through not only just physical stress but also emotional stresses. The emotional stresses are there. It is definitely evident in one drop of blood. It can be seen, and if our treatments, which are nutritional treatments—what we eat, what we drink, how we live, if and how we exercise—can make an impact, then it can be verified in the blood. And yet who's looking at it? So what we're looking at is how do we manage not only our physical body, but also our emotional body.

REVERSING CANCER

"As a chemist trained to interpret data, it is incomprehensible to me that physicians can ignore the clear evidence that chemotherapy does much, much more harm than good."
Alan C. Nixon, Ph.D., Past President,
American Chemical Society

I would like to start out by just having you read a letter that was sent to me recently. As you read, think of someone who may be having a similar challenge regardless of where it is in the body. Here's the letter:

In June of 2005, my wife had breast cancer, the right breast. Surgery, micro-calcification and a lumpectomy, 2.7 mm tumor. She had an OncoDx DNA test and the score said she had a low chance of reoccurrence. So she didn't need chemo but she did do radiation. We started the alkaline program at the end of June '05 and continue today. We both have had tremendous improvements in our health, thanks to you. February of 2006, instead of yearly mammograms we asked for a sonogram. Nothing showed up but somehow was talked into a mammogram and they found a micro-calcification in her other breast, the left breast. Based on the best information I could find, we refused a needle biopsy and more mammograms. Of course, the doctors thought we were crazy but said they would monitor her. We asked for an MRI but I found out they use a toxic metal, gadolinium for contrast for the digital images. So we don't know what to do at this point except follow the pH program. It's not that I doubt that it works because it makes more sense than anything I've come across. But it's a serious matter. Kim is my sole mate and wife for 23 years. pH has been good. Morning urine 7.5 to 8. Saliva has decreased from 7 down to 6.5. I'm not sure why. We are taking a colon cleanse product and probiotic per microscopist suggestion. I'm not sure if that's anything to do with it. Later during the day the pH is 8 to 9. Saliva is 7 to 8. Recently we attended the Cancer Control Society seminar and had our blood tested. The microscopist mentioned above was very impressed with our blood and asked us what we were doing. He said he had never seen a couple with results that were so identical. He did find some yeast in my wife's blood so we were trying to fine-tune the program along with his suggestions. pH Miracle doing real salt, magnesium 800 mg, sodium bicarbonate, glutathione, zinc, vitamin D, E, B complex and a high energy multi-vitamin, juicing greens and green mix and exercise.

Here are my questions:

1. *What would you recommend for your wife if she was in this situation?*
2. *Would you do a needle biopsy or more mammograms?*
3. *Is it necessary to monitor her calcification and breast?*
4. *She does blood work every three months, is that good enough?*

Now as you're thinking about these questions, you could rephrase this for a man; what would you recommend for your husband if he was in a similar situation? Would you do a biopsy or maybe some other types of prostate tests like a PSA test? Is it necessary to monitor calcifications in and around the tissue, the bladder or otherwise? Does having blood work done every three months, is that enough?

Looking at those questions, it's interesting that as we understand the foundational principle of what cancer is—ie, not a cell but a liquid—and as we understand that liquid is flowing through our bodies and is produced as a waste product of metabolism—a waste product of cell transformation—as energy is being consumed as cells break down. As food breaks down, acids are created. These acids are highly toxic and they come in over a thousand different compounds. Some of them we are familiar with like ethanol alcohol, lactic acid, uric acid or nitric acid. We're familiar with many of these compounds. If these acids, these toxins are not properly eliminated through urination, perspiration, respiration or defecation, then the acid catchers, which are the connective tissues—our muscles—actually uptake these acids, these toxins, to maintain and preserve the integrity of the blood which is the most important organ of the human body. The blood has to be maintained at its delicate pH balance of 7.365 at the cost of all other tissue. This is a flowing living organ and without it there would be no life. So everything is compromised in order to maintain the delicate pH balance of those fluids. We can measure these fluids on a daily basis.

There is a lot of mention in this letter about pH. And just like the ocean has ebbs and tides, we find that during the afternoon, particularly around 2:00 p.m. in the afternoon, our pH is at the highest. We find that in a 24-hour period the pH is at its lowest at 2:00 a.m. in the morning. So we have times during the afternoon as we noticed in this letter that the pHs were running between 8 and 9. Where earlier in the morning the pHs were running in the 7 and 8's. In some cases, the saliva may be getting down into the 6's. It's critical that we maintain our pH of our saliva, all of our fluids, our sweat, our urine; even our defecations should have a pH of 7.2 or better. And we can monitor these fluids throughout the day. It's more difficult to monitor the pH of the blood of course, and it's very much constant. This is why it is not part of a traditional type of blood chemistry test or blood test. They very seldom will test the pH because it's so constant. But any variation moving from 7.365 and up indicates the body is in preservation mode.

This is why it's so important when we're doing a test, especially in the case of cancer that we ask our doctor as part of a panel that they do a pH of blood, because if the pH is in the 7.40 and above then we know that our body is in preservation, we're in a state of tissue acidosis. We can actually corroborate that particular test with our urine because generally, the patient who has cancer, will also show if they have adequate reserves, an increase in the pH, or when we're in a serious degeneration, we'll see that the pH has dropped in the 5's. This is an indication of tissue acidosis and the same thing happens as the pH of the blood moves up, that is an indication for the blood that the body is in preservation mode, and we are in a state of latent tissue or tissue acidosis. This will also once again be indicated by the pH of the urine, which will also show generally speaking in the 5's. We need to move that pH up as quickly as possible because the urine is not an indicator of the blood pH but of the tissue pH. For it is the elimination of the toxins that are coming out of the tissues that are being urinated out from the blood and therefore it is a direct indication of tissue acidosis. So it is very important to monitor that—and the ideal pH of the urine is 7.2 or better. If we have any condition that is cancerous, and you've probably heard me say this before, the cancer conditions are a systemic problem that localizes at the weakest part of the body, not a localized problem that metastasized.

We can monitor at home. It is definitely preventative. By monitoring the pH, maintaining the delicate pH balance of the fluids of the body at

7.2 or better, if we are seeing anything less than that, then we can use alkalizing doses of sodium bicarbonate, potassium bicarbonate, magnesium bicarbonate, calcium bicarbonate, what I call the four very powerful salts that we can use to begin the alkalizing process. If you'll take a scoop of just sodium bicarbonate or if you have a compounding pharmacist—so you can ask them to put together a mixture of equal parts of sodium and potassium bicarbonate—then you can take a scoop (which would be approximately two teaspoons of the mixture), put it in about three to four ounces of distilled or purified water. Now you can drink that and within 30 minutes, your urine will go from a state of acidity to a state of alkalinity. You will also want to begin the hydration process as well. After you have that three to four ounces of highly alkalizing substance, then you want to follow that up with your green drink because that is critically important to continue the hydration—as you begin to saturate your tissues like a sponge with alkalinity.

You want to saturate the tissues with alkalinity, because when we're dealing with cancer, what precedes the cancerous tissue is the formation of fibrous materials that cross link to form the tumor as a protective mechanism to protect the tissues, the healthy tissues from fermentation of acid, which is the only cause of tissue breakdown. There's other adjuncts to that that can contribute to it, but the major contributor to tissue fermentation breakdown is our own waste products that have not been properly eliminated, so the body goes into preservation mode, like we mentioned earlier, and begins to pull calcium ions from the blood and from the bone to help neutralize or buffer these metabolic acids in order to protect the body from spoiling.

This is the reason why you find micro-calcifications in the breasts. There is no problem with a micro-calcification in the breast. No one has ever died from a micro-calcification in the brain or the breast or in the prostate for that matter. But they do die from acids tenderizing and fermenting and rotting the tissues. So the body goes into preservation mode to neutralize those acids. If we are finding micro-calcifications, this is the indication that we are at a state of late tissue acidosis, nothing more, nothing less. There is no need to do any further testing. We already know that the signs are there. We can know that through testing urine. We can know that through sonograms which are less harmful than mammograms or MRI's or CAT scans, which use radioactive isotopes that literally poison our bodies with radiation or radiated sugar, which provides even more acidity and more toxins that the body has to deal with.

> Case in Point: Ever since mammograms were introduced, the incidence of ductal carcinoma in situ (DCIS), a type of breast cancer, has increased by 328%! At least 200% of this increase is attributed to the harmful radiation of mammograms.

Once we have these symptomatic markers, maybe it is a PSA, if the PSA is showing above a normal marker of 4 or 5, generally current allopathic medicine would want to do a biopsy, but there is no need for a biopsy, for this would be like opening Pandora's Box, disturbing the tissue. The body is in preservation mode. The increase of specific antigens in the blood, CA-125 or whatever test we're doing is an indication that our body is in latent tissue acidosis—and we need to begin the alkalizing process. This is also substantiated with the pH in saliva and urine or sweat for that matter or even our bowel eliminations that are less than what would be normal: 7.2 or above. As we begin the alkalizing process, we can see the changes that will take place.

So what would I recommend if my wife were in such situation with micro-calcifications? I would allow the body to continue to do what it's doing but to support it with an alkalizing lifestyle and diet. The focus is not in treating the tissue. The focus is in changing the lifestyle and the diet which incorporates the basic tenants as outlined in the pH Miracle for Weight Loss, Chapter 11. The seven steps to ideal incredible health. The seven steps in preventing or *reversing* cancerous tissue. Because remember what we said earlier, there is no cancer, there are just states of balance or imbalance and there is no such thing as a cancer cell. Because cancer is not a noun. It is a description. It is an adjective describing what has happened to the cell. So cancer is a liquid. And tumor is nothing more than the body's way of protecting itself. Protecting healthy tissue. Metastasis is only localized acidity spoiling other cells much like a rotten apple spoiling a bushel of healthy apples.

These are things that help us to understand a better approach than chemical therapy or radiation, because here radiation or surgery is focused on the tissue, not on the environment. Like the woman who wrote the letter, you can take the right breast off but there's still another breast in which the body can throw acids which can then throw the body into preservation mode forming micro-calcifications. In the case of brain cancer, in brain tissue, micro-calcifications always precede the fermentation of the tissue and the formation of the tumor. The tumor being the solution to the problem.

We don't need any tests to determine that this is cancerous or non-cancerous. It is the body in its perfect way trying to protect itself against our own lifestyle and dietary choices. We are experiencing the consequence of *choice*. And a little indulgence, well it's only one piece of chocolate or it's only one glass of milk or it's only one piece of pie or whatever the rationalization; for someone who's been in a state of imbalance, there is no going back to an inverted way of living, eating and thinking—provided one wants to protect themselves from having a reoccurrence.

So the questions, *what would I suggest to my wife?* I would say begin the program 100% with no variation as it pertains to those foods which are alkalizing. So where are those foods listed? They are listed in the book, *The pH Miracle for Weight Loss*. Never cross the line to the acidic foods. Read that book, which I like to call *The pH Miracle for Everything*, because it incorporates everything that you need to know from not only just the physical aspects of alkalizing the body, but also from the emotional and spiritual aspects too. The micro-calcifications need no further research. There is no need for biopsy. There is no more need for mammograms. There is a great need for change—to get different results. Now as far as monitoring this, we don't need more testing as it pertains to MRI's and CAT scans or mammograms. What we need is to monitor the pH of the fluids, and this is the most inexpensive way for us to monitor our health.

As far as the blood tests, the expansion on those CA's if we want to do a CEA in the case of prostate cancer, or a PSA, all these different acronyms—and there are many—to monitor these acidic markers called antigens that are showing up in the blood, the cancer antigens, the prostate antigens, this is an indication of tissue acidosis where the body needs more alkalinity. I've never seen a case where those markers are not reversed, if not completely eliminated, if one is willing to follow the program 100%. Because what I am going to say right now is critically important: *All cancerous tissue is curable.* Not all patients are. I'll say it one more time. *All cancerous tissue is preventable, reversible, curable, but not all patients are because they are not willing to do what it takes to bring their body in balance.* They are not willing to give up the tobacco. They're not willing to give up that drink or that one glass of wine. They're not willing to give up the coffee, the tea, the goji berries, the chocolate… whatever it is that's keeping an individual back from extraordinary and incredible health, energy and vitality. They're not getting up to the six liters of green drinks. They're not monitoring every fluid of their body, every time they urinate. They're not monitoring their saliva five minutes before they eat, five minutes after. And they're not monitoring the blood on a regular basis to make sure that one is moving in the right direction. Doing everything possible and probably the most critical one is to move from fear which is false evidence appearing real to faith which is the first attribute in thinking healthy. Faith is what heals. Fear is what kills.

There is new research showing that vegetables will actually prevent brain degeneration where fruits will not. People say… well why did God create this fruit? Well let me tell you why fruit is created. In fact, everything God has created serves to give us the experience of duality, and through that experience of duality, and through free agency, we might choose between good and evil, right and wrong, health or sickness, so that we may gain knowledge. That cancerous tissue by any name is nothing more than the consequence of choice. It's not something one gets. Someone doesn't get prostate cancer. You have to work on it every day. Someone doesn't get breast cancer or brain cancer. You have to work on it every day.

So the formula for preventing or reversing cancer, which was our first question, is understanding that the human organism is alkaline by design and every fluid in the body is alkaline. Everything that we put in the body should be supporting that alkaline pH, with no exception. No rationalization. And if I have a cancerous diagnosis, I know of no reason on this good planet earth as to how chemotherapy could actually contribute to the alkaline design of the human organism. Just as a banana rots and changes, as that tissue deteriorates and becomes sweeter and sweeter because sugar, and again I want you to listen to this carefully, sugar is a waste product of cellular degeneration. It's an acid. That's why bananas get sweet. That's why sugar is attracted. Especially radioactive sugar and MRI's are attracted to this environment, this waste, because cancer cells live within their own waste products. Secondary metabolites like acetaldehyde which if we dilute it we can call it vinegar. God only knows why health professionals recommend it as if it's something good for the body. It's actually like putting kerosene on a fire.

We have to be very clear about everything that we put into our mouth as a reflection of everything that we put into our minds, we have to be able to manage our thoughts, our words and our deeds. This is not an easy thing. As I'm speaking to you, I must tell you I also speak to myself. We have to be diligent and committed with certainty moving forward in faith in order to obtain the fruit of the tree of life which is most desirous above all things. Which is life itself. Yet it is so simple it eludes most of us, because we don't understand this foundational principle—that the human organism is alkaline by design and acidic by function. That eating for example is an acidic function. That's why people who eat less, not all the time but generally, create less acidity and are many more times healthier than people that are over eating. Now science is saying there is a factor of obesity as one of the conditions that leads to cancer. Well diabetes too. These are just progressive steps to the fermenting banana. But when the banana becomes rotten, there are times when surgery is necessary.

We need to cut out the rotten tissue just as we would take a rotten apple out of a bushel of healthy apples, especially if the tumor does not complete its formation and encapsulation, because a tumor goes from something very pliable to something very, very hard. That's the difference between malignancy and non-malignancy. One has blood, life flowing to it. It hasn't completely encapsulated. And that which has been encapsulated by the fiber monomers completely walling it away from any blood whatsoever, becomes crystallized and hard. No one ever dies from a tumor. They die from states of over acidity. I want you to understand that. I want you to believe it. It is true. With all my heart I know this. I know it as a scientist but I also know it on a spiritual level too. No one has ever died from a tumor. They died from localized systemic poisoning of their own waste products from their own doing. Medical science needs to wake up to this.

So there are inexpensive ways to prevent a reverse cancer. I mean how inexpensive is sodium bicarbonate? How quickly can you settle an acidic or an upset stomach by simply taking a scoop, two or three teaspoons of sodium bicarbonate or potassium bicarbonate, putting it into distilled or better yet ionized alkaline water and drinking three or four ounces of that to settle the acid of the stomach—to re-alkalize that alkaline environment. Yes, you've probably heard this for the first time. This is not taught in any textbooks. You won't find it in the traditional biology books. You won't find it in any alternative books. The stomach is *alkaline* by design. The purpose of the stomach is not to digest food, in that it is not an organ of digestion but an organ of contribution and its main purpose is to produce sodium bicarbonate. From the cover cells, it releases bicarbonate, it's an alkaline environment. It's alkaline by design. And the pH of the stomach should range anywhere from 7.2 or up, not 1.5 to 3 which is currently taught in both traditional and non-traditional medicine.

There are lots of natural treatments, which we'll talk about later on. As we look at the seven steps to our pH Miracle for health, energy and vitality, to remove the acids that are spoiling our bodies, the first step is to super hydrate with alkaline fluids. The second is eat right for your life. This is a *choice*. Next is exercise, yes we need to pee our way to health but we also need to *sweat our way to health*. If you're not moving, you're dying. Exercise needs to happen every day. There will never be a drug or surgery that will ever fix problems due to lack of exercise. The fourth step is you need to know the types of supplements you're taking are alkaline and alkalizing to the fluids of the body. You need to understand that our emotions are so powerful and create several thousand times more acids than our metabolic wastes. That our thoughts are so powerful and demand so much energy to carry out. That as we're in our thoughts, these thoughts create acids that will spoil our body. The sixth step is to set goals—we need to write them down.

One of the goals that I would suggest you do on a regular basis—and to start this goal you have to make a small purchase of some litmus paper or some pH paper—and then get a diary and start recording your pH, graphing this out, both for urine and saliva. Every time before you eat, five minutes before, you test your saliva and five minutes after you test your saliva and you write it down. You keep score. Anytime that your urine or your saliva or your sweat is below 7.2, you take an alkalizing dose of bi-salts or tri-salts or quad salts, depending on what your compounding pharmacist will put together for you, to begin this alkalizing process. It's the best chemical therapy and yes, sodium bicarbonate is a chemical, it's a compound of sodium and carbon, bicarbonate. It is HCO_3 but it is inexpensive. It is an alkalizing compound. It will not hurt or destroy healthy tissue.

Of course the seventh step, which is cleanse your body from the inside out, could actually be the first step. It probably should be the first step for those who have a serious fermentation state or a state of imbalance, where we begin this entire program on a baby food diet or a liquefied or juiced diet. The purpose of that is obvious, when we realize that everything has to be liquefied or pureed in an alkaline state anyway before it leaves the stomach. We might as well prepare the food in that state so that we're not using a lot of energy which creates even more acid to break down our foods that we're eating. We don't want to spend a lot of time and energy wasted on breakdown, we'll let the juicers and the mixers and blenders do all of that, so that we can have a predigested food that is all ready to be utilized by the body. That just takes some getting used to, but you started out that way. I don't know if you remember, you started out on liquid foods for the first three, six, nine months. When you're in a state of imbalance you get to go back to that state again. It is very, very healthy. You can do it for an indefinite period of time. There is no need for us to eat solid food because it always has to be liquefied and alkalized before it leaves the stomach, before it enters into the duodenum and then into the small intestine—the pH of that food should be at least 8.2 to 8.4. Highly alkalized, ready to be transformed into new blood.

This is why these good folks who had their blood tested by a microscopist, their blood looks so consistent. Because you are what you eat and you are what you drink. That is a reflection of the blood because the blood is a reflection of you. It is who you are. It is your identity. The blood is uniquely you. It is the life of your body. The best way to get that healthy as it has been defined, the first nutrition that's defined in all the writings in history are actually defined by Moses in Genesis Chapter 1: Verse 28-30. It tells us the specific foods that we should eat, and specifically by color—and the color is green. All green foods should be for your meat. It is going back to the Garden of Eden.

72

It is going back to the grasses. It is going back to the vegetables, the spinach, the broccoli, the cucumbers. All of the alkalizing low sugar fruits, green fruits and all the alkalizing vegetables.

With regard to exercise, it's not only important to exercise but it is important to exercise properly. You have to move the body because, when the body is moving, that's the way to move acids out of the tissues and out through the pores of the skin or out then back into blood circulation and filtered out through the kidneys. So the most important thing that you can do while you're exercising is sweating. If you're not sweating, you're not exercising properly, and that's a concern. There's something you can do to increase sweating and that's increase hydration. Your body uses between 2 ½ to 3 liters a day, just for normal functioning. You loose that much. So you need to replace that fluid every day at least three liters. But on top of that if you have a cancerous condition, you have to get up into the pH miracle zone, and the pH miracle zone is a minimum of 4 to 6 liters. In serious conditions you could be up to as many as 8 to 12 liters. We have a client patient in New Zealand who was diagnosed with melanoma. In fact, four of his friends were diagnosed at the same time and they're dead and he is the only one alive. He was drinking between 8 to 12 liters a day of fluids in order to saturate the tissues so he could move those acids out of the tissues. So you've got to create the hydration in order to move the toxins.

I find for most folks, that the more that they drink, the thirstier they get. Sometimes the patient is so sick that we have to involve their doctor to hook them up to an IV of saline solution and sodium bicarbonate. That is one of the very simple and inexpensive treatments that can be done simply by the medical doctor. No toxic chemicals but simply an IV of 1% saline solution and 8 to 10% solution of sodium bicarbonate per liter, which is very simple to do. In fact, it's interesting, anyone that is in any type of toxemia, or where the pH is dropping and this is of course the case in cancerous conditions, prior to it going up and the body going into body waste, this is how you prevent body wasting, particularly in a cancerous situation, is you maintain the alkaline design of the fluids of the body. You cannot let it drop below that 7.2—this is the simplest way to do it. So you can hook yourself up to 3 to 4 to 5 to 6 liters in one day. This is actually very helpful and very hydrating to the body and it helps to move a lot of the

73

acidity that's been taken up by the acid catchers—the connective tissues—that need to be flushed. It also helps to saturate the tissues in alkalinity in preparation for the body to then release that acidity via the vital lymphatic system through the pores of the skin through sweat or back into circulation through urination.

There are some other things that we can do in one of our other steps and that's of course we need to use alkalizing foods and alkalizing supplements. If the food and supplements we consume do not change, the concern I have is that our outer ecology is going to worsen. And if doctors don't change their minds about nutrition, I'm concerned man as a biological part of this earth will soon be extinct. Our intestines must be healed. Our bowels need to be healed. There is a connection. I call it the five B's. The five B's is base diet, healthy bowels, healthy blood, healthy brain, healthy body. It's base, bowels, blood, brain and body. So if our bowels are not healthy, our brain cannot be healthy. Neither can our blood. Neither can our body. Our intestines must be healed since they are as polluted as the streams and rivers and lakes and our oceans. From a good earth, one regenerates one's health. Our blood is but an agent of this earth and you've heard it in the good book, "from dust we are and from dust we will return." Because we truly are becoming what we eat, what we drink and what we think.

I've got six powerful nutrients: these are the super antioxidants—the super antacids—and they need to be taken in combination with a healthy alkalizing diet and hydration. The first one is acetylcarnitine (ALC), 200 milligrams six times a day. B3, niacin 25 milligrams six times a day, conjugated unsaturated fats, conjugated linoleic acids, omega 6's and omega 3's. You should be taking between 2,000 and 3,000 milligrams six to nine times a day. Co-enzyme Q1 and co-enzyme Q-10, 800 milligrams daily. N-acetyl cysteine (NAC), which is actually the backbone and precursor to glutathione, 1,500 milligrams six to nine times a day. And the granddaddy of them all, glutathione's sulfhydryl or GSH as it's known, 1,200 milligrams six to nine times a day. For those who are not familiar with GSH or glutathione, it's a peptide that occurs naturally within the body. It's called a tri-peptide because it has three amino acids: L-cysteine, L-glutamate and L-glycine. When the cells have enough L-cysteine, and that's why you take both of them together, this is when GSH can be formed. Without it, it cannot be formed.

So without L-cysteine, the cells of the body cannot protect themselves from acid. It is the major antacid in which the organized blood and the organized tissue protects itself with glutathione. So glutathione is one of the major super antioxidants that helps to detoxify our bodies of excess acidity—thereby supporting the white blood cells which are our garbage collection service. It is a powerful anti-tumor agent because if the body is less acidic, there is less spoiling of cells. And if there is less spoiling of cells, there is less fiber monomers being conjugated up to cross-link and form in a capsulation of these morbid cells.

It also helps in the prevention of malnutrition and the body wasting, because the body wastes itself in order to maintain the constant supply of blood which is life itself. That's why you have to watch on a CBC, that's a comprehensive blood test, you have to watch the red blood cell count. Red blood cell count should be at 5 million per cubic millimeter. If it's greater than that, the body is in preservation mode. If it's less than that, the body is in body wasting. The body is using its own body cells in order to maintain blood. That means we're not eating enough green foods. We're not getting enough green drinks. That's why these good folks in this letter had such good-looking blood because they were drinking and eating greens. That's what you build blood with. It's molecularly identical. It's molecularly correct. The blood of green plants is what builds our blood.

On top of that, when we are building good healthy blood, we build good healthy tissue because all body cells are a product of blood. Skin is a product of blood. Heart is a product of blood. Liver is a product of blood. Everything is a product of blood. So the quality of blood determines the quality of the body tissue. That is why there is a base diet, bowel, blood, brain, body connection because what goes in the bowel determines the quality of the blood and the quality of the blood will determine the quality of the brain. So if you are having cognitive dysfunction, or any dysfunction, physically or emotionally, the problem is in the bowels. And the problem is not in the bowels, the problem goes upstream so you have to go back up in the intestine to the stomach to the esophagus to the mouth. What am I putting in my mouth? Or what am I putting in my brain? In my head? What am I listening to? What am I thinking? We have to go upstream to determine what is going on and we have to evaluate that. Then we need to be accountable. We have to keep score and that's the purpose of keeping a diary.

If you are doing traditional type treatments of chemotherapy and radiation, glutathione will protect you against the side effects of these very toxic protocols. So what I suggest (and you need to clear this with your doctor before you do anything, I'm not telling you what to do, I'm just telling you what I would do for myself or my wife) I would take 1,200 milligrams six to nine times daily orally. If I was really aggressive I would take 1,200 milligrams per one liter of 1% saline solution four times a day by IV. On top of that I'd probably take 25 mills or 600 milligrams and put it in a nebulizer and just breathe it in, because it goes directly into the blood stream. But if I don't have a nebulizer and I don't have a doctor who's willing to hook me up to an IV, because they're living in a state of fear, then what I should do is take the 1,200 milligrams, six to nine times a day in a capsulated form. And if I can find it conjugated, it's very expensive if you can find it, I would take it in a liquefied form. With that I would take 500 milligrams six to nine times of N-acetyl cysteine (NAC). These are the super antacids, antioxidants that will actually begin the process of bringing your body back to the state of balance. You can check it by monitoring your pH of your urine and saliva. Then on top of that, looking at the live blood to see how the blood is organizing itself and to look at the context to see the cleanliness of that environment and how it's changing—how the blood is coagulating—or to go back to your doctor and have another CEA or CA125 or a PSA or whatever the test or marker that you're currently having your doctor do. These can be monitored. This is not a problem, and it's not that invasive to take a vial of blood and to test for some of these markers.

But you'll notice that when you do this, the markers will be going down because you're now doing what is right. You're following a course that's bringing the body back to a state of alkalinity, and you're starting to understand that the body runs on energy—electricity—it doesn't run on food, it doesn't run on calories, it doesn't run on carbohydrates or fats or proteins. It runs on electrons, and the more electrical energy you can put in your body, the healthier you are going to be. And the more chlorophyll that you can put in the body and the good healthy fats, the healthier your blood is going to be and that's going to equate into healthy tissue.

You see how easy this all is? We don't need to make it that much more difficult.

INSULIN POTENTIATION THERAPY (IPT)

Pharmaceutical drugs and medical treatments such as chemotherapy are examples of therapies which not only harm good cells but also shut down the body's immune system at a time when the body needs it most.

This happens because chemotherapy agents (ie, poisons known as cytotoxic drugs) do not discriminate between cancer cells and other normal cells in the patient's body. They kill both kinds of cells, especially the fast growing cells in your intestines, bombarding them with the same chemical weapon. That's why all chemotherapy patients feel like hell and

most wish they were dead!

According to an article in the January, 2003 issue of *Life Extension*, *"the institutions we have counted on to find a cure (National Cancer Institute, American Cancer Society, drug companies, etc.) have failed. This is not an allegation, but an admission made by the National Cancer Institute itself."*

Knowledge is power. If your doctor won't cooperate with you in considering other gentler alternatives, you should get another doctor.

If you are still considering conventional chemotherapy, despite there being many alternative treatments like the pH Miracle for Cancer by Dr. Robert O. Young discussed in this book, here is some detail on an option.

IPT is Insulin Potentiation Therapy, a strategic use of the same natural hormone diabetics use—insulin—to dramatically improve effectiveness and delivery of chemotherapy.

When a doctor administers Insulin Potentiation Chemotherapy (IPT), also known as low dose chemotherapy, the first thing he or she does is to gently lower the patient's blood sugar level with insulin. The cancer cells, because they must have sugar to live, become ravenous and open those insulin receptors wide to get at whatever they can find in the blood stream's diminishing supply. When the blood sugar level has dropped enough, the doctor will administer a low dose of chemotherapy. The cancer cells, having 10-20 times more insulin receptors on their surface than normal cells, take it all in.

And because insulin assists in the delivery of the drugs, IPT uses about 90% less chemotherapy compared to the normal "high dose" chemotherapy and results in far fewer side effects. This means that patients continue to thrive, maintain their lifestyle, and be vital while the cancer is eradicated.

Another major advantage is that the patient retains much more energy to apply other healing methods such as the pH Miracle lifestyle and diet program. Here is a quote from a popular IPT web site:

"Conventional chemotherapy treatment can be so taxing that patients won't even consider, let alone take action on, other cancer-fighting measures such as diet modification, exercise and meditation."

To find out more about this treatment and locate an IPT doctor near you, go to:
http://www.IPTforcancer.com

For some testimonials and other information about IPT, go to:
http://www.iptq.com

PH MIRACLE RECIPES

"Those who think they have no time for healthy eating will sooner or later have to find time for illness."
Edward Stanley, Author of *The Conduct of Life*

"The doctor of the future will no longer treat the human frame with drugs, but rather will cure and prevent disease with nutrition."
Thomas Edison, American inventor and scientist

All that you've read to this point wouldn't get you very far without this chapter, which provides the secret to putting this plan into action: delicious recipes for alkaline food. Understanding why it is important to stop eating acidifying foods, and wanting to do so, is all well and good, but then the question remains: what <u>are</u> you going to eat? Look no further for the answer. And: get your taste buds ready for a treat. They may be dulled currently to the exquisite wonder of nature's bounty, but soon after you switch over to this way of eating they'll be alive to every natural, wholesome flavor it has to offer.

Our first book, The pH Miracle, contains an extensive recipe section as well, so if you ever exhaust what's here you have an option for more ideas about eating in harmony with the pH miracle plan. And we hope *you* will improvise and innovate as you grow more comfortable with preparing food the pH Miracle way.

In this chapter, you'll find sections for Drinks and Shakes; Soups; Salads; Dressings, Dips and Sauces; Entrees/Side dishes and Snacks/Desserts. Recipes marked with an asterisk (*) are suitable for use in a liquid feast.

> **NB: The most important thing for you to remember as you begin to prepare your food is that cancer cells absolutely love sugar—and sugar feeds cancer. That's right, sugar is the food of cancer with a cancer cell having 96 sugar receptors compared to a normal cell with 4! So steer clear of all acidic foods and beverages that cancer cells love.**

DRINKS AND SHAKES

Many of these drinks and shakes can serve as a complete meal. They enter the bloodstream quickly and give the greatest amount of concentrated nutrition and energy with the least amount of digestive stress of anything you could eat.

The Raw Perfection Morning Monster Juice. Serves 1.
(Donated by Mike Nash)

This is great when you need something that's gonna stick with you until mid-day; the fat will help you feel full. Besides providing that fat, the avocado is the key to the creaminess of this smoothie.

 1 package (bunch) kale
 1 head of celery
 1 lemon
 A handful of spinach leaves
 1 avocado
 1 scoop of green powder
 1 chili pepper

Put kale, celery and lemon through juicer, then combine in blender with remaining ingredients.

AvoRado Kid Super Green Shake*. Serves 1.

This is by far our favorite cool green shake, and we've enjoyed it for breakfast, lunch and dinner, or anytime we want a snack. It's a great way to get the concentrated nutrition and chlorophyll of green powder and soy sprouts powder (and an especially great way to get it into your kids). The cucumber and lime cool the body, and the essential fats in God's great butter, avocado, and the soy sprouts make this shake one that you can burn on for many hours.

 1 avocado
 ½ English cucumber
 1 tomatillo
 1 lime (peeled)
 2 cups fresh spinach
 2 scoops soy sprouts powder

1 scoop of green powder
1 pkg. stevia
6-8 ice cubes

Blend in a blender on high speed to a thick, smooth consistency. Serve immediately.

Variations:

* Add 1 tsp. of almond butter for a nuttier flavor.
*Add coconut milk or fresh silky almond milk for a creamier shake.
*Make a parfait by layering the shake with layers of dehydrated unsweetened coconut and sprinkle some of the coconut on top.
*Substitute a grapefruit or lemon for the lime for a different taste.
*add 1 Tbs fresh grated ginger
*Add some seasonings that are bottled in oil (without alcohol) for a new exciting twist of flavor.

In the summer, freeze AvoRado Kid into pops for a cool frozen treat. You can also completely freeze and then partially thaw small portions of the shake, then chop it up to enjoy as a slush.

Very Veggie Shake. Serves 2
(Donated by Parvin Moshiri)

1 c. distilled water
¼ cup flax seed oil or olive oil
2 small cucumbers, sliced
1 cup spinach
2 avocados
1/3 head of Romaine lettuce
½ cup Broccoli
¼ cup cilantro
¼ cup parsley
2 stalks of celery cut into pieces
1/8 cup fresh mint leaves (or 1 tsp. dry)
2 medium limes or 1 lemon
1/8 cup fresh dill (optional)

Place water in a blender then add oil. Turn blender on and add remaining ingredients one at a time. When everything is chopped up, turn up blender to "liquefy" until you get a beautiful smooth and creamy green shake.

Zesty Lemon Ginger Shake. Serves 1.
(Donated by Karen Rose)

This refreshing shake can help raise blood sugar levels quickly.

  1 lemon, peeled and chopped
  2 T chopped fresh ginger
  1 avocado
  1 small cucumber
  1-2 t Soft tofu

Mix all ingredients together in the blender until creamy (add water if necessary for desired consistency).

Variation:

To make this higher in protein as well as even more lemony, add:

  1 lemon or lime
  2 scoops soy sprouts powder
  1 scoop green powder
  2 pkg stevia (with fiber)
  ¼ c soft tofu
  6-8 ice cubes

Paul's Breakfast in a Blender. Serves 1.
(Donated by Paul A. Repicky, Ph.D.)

This is a *chewy* sort of breakfast (or anytime) shake which will keep you going for hours.

  ½ large, non-sweet grapefruit (or, 1 small one), outer layer of rind peeled off (the white inner rind is quite nutritious) and core and seeds removed
  handful of sprouts (alfalfa, or clover, or other)
  handful of fresh spinach
  1/3 c fresh ground flax seed
  1-2 Tbs. UDO's Oil
  2 cups broccoli
  ½ English cucumber
  1 ½ cups water

Mix all ingredients in blender on medium speed (or higher if you like it smoother).

Adjust quantities to taste; this usually makes 32-34 ounces.

Minty Mock Malt. Serves 2.
(Donated by Matthew and Ashley Rose Lisonbee)

½ English cucumber
juice of 1 lime
juice of 1 grapefruit
1 avocado
1 cup raw spinach
½ can coconut milk
1 t green powder
2 t soy sprouts powder
8-10 drops pH drops
2-4 sprigs for fresh mint leaves or ½ t mint flavoring (no alcohol)
(Frontier brand)
14 ice cubes

Combine all ingredients in a blender and blend to desired consistency.

Variation: leave out the ice cubes, and freeze malt into pops.

Chi's Green Drink. Serves 2.
(Donated by Jill Butler)

1 head Romaine or Boston lettuce. Use the greenest leafy parts, omitting the really light green stems if you wish.
3 cloves of garlic
1 lemon
¾ cup water
½ cup olive oil
1 piece of cut fresh ginger (optional)
dash of sea salt
dash of cayenne pepper
a combination of all or one or none of the following:
basil leaves
parsley
watercress (leaves only)
1 cucumber, peeled
a little steamed broccoli
(or use whatever combination of green veggies you like.
Experiment!)

Blend in blender until smooth.

Carrot Crunch. Serves 1.
(Donated by Randy Wakefield)

This helps raise low blood sugar.

 1/2 t green powder
 7 drops pH drops
 1 cup fresh carrot juice
 1 chopped carrot
 4 ice cubes

Combine ingredients in electric or hand blender and blend until smooth. Serve sprinkled with nutmeg.

Fresh Silky Almond Milk. Serves 4-6; makes appx. 1 quart.

4 cups of fresh raw almonds
Pure water
nylon stocking (for straining)

Soak 4 cups of fresh raw almonds over night in a bowl of water. Drain. Place the almonds into a blender until it is a third full (about two cups), then add pure water to fill the blender up. Blend on high speed until you have a white creamy looking milk. Take a nylon stocking, (I use a (clean!) white knee high nylon stocking) and pour the mixture through it over a bowl or pan, and let it drain. Squeeze with your hand to get the last of the milk through the nylon. Thin with water to desired consistency.

Drink as is, or add a bit of stevia to sweeten it. Or, use in soups, shakes or puddings. Almond milk will stay fresh for about 3 days in the refrigerator.

(Use the solids you strained out with the stocking in the shower for a great body scrub)

Soups

Soups are especially great for cancer patients because, since they are liquid, they provide energy, chlorophyll and hydration as you recover from this condition.

Think of soup as a breakfast food, now that you are avoiding the conventional starchy, sugar, and high protein options.

Navy Bean Soup. Serves 2-4
(Donated by Roxy Boelz)

3rd Place, pH Miracle Recipe Contest

This soup will help raise low blood sugar levels.

  1 cup aduki beans, soaked overnight
  1 cup navy beans, soaked overnight
  1 small onion, chopped
  2 large carrots, grated
  Real Salt to taste
  2 t fresh ginger, grated
  1 cup celery, chopped
  Nutmeg or cardamom

Cook the beans till just tender. Cool slightly. If necessary, add water to get the consistency of soup you want. Add salt, onion, carrots and ginger. Transfer to food processor or blender and process to the texture desired. You can add celery with the ingredients to be blended, or afterwards for crunchiness. Serve sprinkled with nutmeg or cardamom or a spice of your choice.

Tortilla Soup*. Serves 2
(Donated by Cheri Freeman)

3rd place, pH Miracle Recipe Contest

This entry won in the "transitional" category. Some people like to use organic chicken broth instead of veggie. This soup, sans tortillas and tofu, would be great for a liquid feast.

  3 cups yeast-free vegetable broth
  1 cup pureed fresh tomatoes or packaged strained tomatoes with
  no preservatives or additives
  8 oz baked seasoned tofu, sliced or coarsely chopped
  olive oil
  2 T garlic, chopped
  2 jalapenos, seeded and chopped very fine
  ½ c. cilantro, chopped very fine
  ½ onion, chopped very fine
  Real Salt to taste
  Garlic pepper blend to taste

1 avocado, diced
sprouted grain tortillas (1/2 for each serving) (optional)

Preheat oven to 200° F. Place your tortilla/s directly on the baking rack until they are crisp Pour your broth and tomato puree in a saucepan and begin heating on very low heat while preparing vegetables and tofu. In a small skillet, brown tofu in olive oil. Add to broth. Add garlic and spices. When warmed, turn off heat, and add avocado to soup. Serve topped with broken bits of tortilla sprinkled on top for some added crunch.

Vegan Chili. Serves 2-4.
(Donated by Cheri Freeman)

Great on cold nights!

3rd place, pH Miracle Recipe Contest [transitional foods]

2 veggie burger patties or crumbles
¼ cup olive oil
½ onion, chopped
1 jalapeno (with or without seeds, depending on how hot you want it)
1 Tbs. Chili powder
1 tsp. Real Salt
2 cloves garlic chopped
3 cups strained tomatoes
2 cups tossed salad (mixed chopped greens, red and yellow peppers, carrots, etc.)
vegan cheese shreds (optional)

In a saucepan or cast iron pot, brown crumbled patties in olive oil. Add all remaining ingredients except salad. Adjust seasonings to your own taste. If you don't like it too hot, you can seed your jalapeno. Put about half of the chili in a blender, add salad mix and puree. Pour back into chili and stir thoroughly. Serve topped with vegan cheese.

French Gourmet Puree. Serves 6.
Donated by Eric Prouty

2nd place, pH Miracle Recipe Contest

This is a beautiful soothing alkaline puree. Sometimes I like to double the amount of lettuce to thin it out a bit.

    1 Avocado
    2 Stalks Celery
    1 Head Romaine Lettuce
    1 Small Tomato
    1 handful Spinach
    1 small Cucumber, peeled
    2 Cloves Garlic
    1/3 Onion
    2 Tbs Olive Oil
    Herbs de Provence
    Sprouts (optional)

Puree all vegetables with a juicer, doing the onion last. Mix in olive oil, and Herbes de Provence to taste. Serve with sprouts sprinkled on top.

Creamy Watercress Soup. Serves 4-6
Donated by Deborah Johnson

    1-cauliflower (cut into 1"pieces)
    2-cups pure water
    2-cups vegetable broth
    2-cups chopped fresh watercress (reserve a sprig or two for garnish)
    1-cup zucchini pieces
    1-cup broccoli pieces
    1-cup celery pieces
    4-green onions, tops removed
    ¼-cup extra virgin olive oil
    Real Salt to taste

Boil water, remove from heat, add cauliflower and allow to rest for 5 minutes. Place cauliflower and water in food processor or blender and process until smooth. Add vegetable broth and remaining ingredients and blend until desired consistency is reached. Do not over blend. Serve warm or chilled. Garnish with a sprig of watercress.

Clean and Simple Soup. Serves 1-2
Donated by Eric Prouty 2nd place winner of Alkalarian recipes, in the pH Miracle Recipe Contest, held by the InnerLight Foundation, July 2003

> 1 Cucumber, cubed
> 1 Avocado, cubed
> mint (optional)

Place ingredients in food processor with S blade. Mix until almost smooth. Serve garnished with mint leaf.

Soothing Cooling Tomato Soup*. Serves 2-4

This silky smooth cooling soup can raise blood sugar if it has dropped too low. The combination of fresh tomatoes and avocado makes it high in lycopene and lucene.

> 6 med. tomatoes juiced and strained (pour through a fine mesh strainer or nylon knee high stocking
> ½ avocado
> ¾ cup fresh coconut water (make sure this is fresh, taken from a coconut)
> 1 cucumber, juiced
> Real Salt to taste
> Stevia (optional)

Blend until smooth. For a sweeter soup, add stevia to taste.

Cool Raw Red Soup. Serves 2-4.
This is a raw soup made by juicing all your veggies and then blending them with avocado and some clear fresh coconut water. It has a cooling effect, and is light and refreshing -- perfect for a hot summer day.

> 1 beet
> ½ large English cucumber
> 4 stalks celery
> 1-2 carrots
> 1 small clove garlic

¼ cup fresh cilantro
½ avocado
¼ cup fresh coconut water (which should be clear and slightly sweet)
Grated veggies (for garnish)

Juice first six ingredients, then pour juice juice through a clean knee high nylon stocking or a fine wire mesh strainer. Mix in blender with avocado and coconut water. Garnish if desired with grated veggies.

Roasted Leek Ginger Soup. Serves 4

Olive or grapeseed oil
1 Cup freshly strained Almond milk
1 leek, thoroughly cleaned and sliced in 1/3 inch slices
1 tsp. fresh ginger cut in thin slices
½ -1 tsp. Real Salt
2 cups Veggie Broth

In a soup pot, stir fry leeks and ginger in oil until softened and browned on edges. Pulse chop leek and ginger in food processor and return to soup pot. Add almond milk, broth and Real Salt. Warm and serve.

Variation: add diced roasted peppers and garlic.

Potato Vegetable Soup. Serves 4
Donated by Terry Douglas

This is a nice full bodied veggie soup that would help raise blood sugar levels.

4-6 small red potatoes
1-2 Tbs. Olive Oil
1 med. Yellow onion, chopped
2 cloves garlic, chopped
2 cans of vegetable stock
1 celery, sliced
2 carrots, sliced into rounds
Salt, Pepper and cayenne
1-2 cups baby spinach leaves
1/2-inch fresh ginger, sliced or julienned

a few leaves of cilantro
½ cucumber chopped
1 tomato chopped
½ green or red pepper, chopped
Bragg Aminos (optional)
Basil (optional)

Cook potatoes in boiling water until tender (about 20 minutes). In a separate soup pan, over low heat, saute onion in olive oil; add garlic when the onion is almost done. Add broth, celery and carrots. If you don't have lots of liquid, add a can of water. Heat until warm, 3-5 minutes. Veggies should still be crunchy. Season to taste with salt, pepper and cayenne. Remove from heat. Add spinach and ginger. To serve, quarter potatoes, and divide into soup bowls. Optional: add a drop of liquid Bragg Aminos and a basil leaf in each bowl. Add soup, and top with cilantro, cucumber, tomatoes and pepper. Serve immediately, with crackers [do you want to refer to another recipe here?] or sliced avocado.

Spicy Latin Lentil Soup. Serves 4
Donated by Cathy Galvis

This cooked soup would help raise blood sugar levels. Buen apetito !

  2 c. lentils
  6 c. water
  2 carrots (sliced)
  1 celery stalk (chopped)
  ½ green pepper (chopped)
  ½ red bell pepper (chopped)
  1 onion (chopped)
  2 cloves garlic (minced)
  2 bay leaves
  1 tsp. Bragg's Amino's
  1 tsp. olive oil
  ½ tsp. jalapeno pepper (seeded and chopped)
  ¼ tsp. cayenne pepper
  1/8 tsp. black pepper
  ¼ c. cilantro (chopped)

In a large pot, add the water and lentils and bring to a boil. Add the carrots, cayenne pepper, black pepper, Braggs and bay leaves. Return to a simmer and cover. In a separate pan, sauté the onions, garlic, green and red peppers, celery and jalapeno pepper in the olive oil for a few minutes. Set aside. Cook the lentils for approximately 20 minutes and add the sautéed onions and peppers. Cook for 10 more minutes, or until the lentils are soft. Serve garnished with the cilantro.

Creamy Cauliflower Confetti Soup

This soup is deceptively creamy-you'd think it had dairy in it. The roasted veggie bits give it, its confetti appearance. Sprinkle roasted bell peppers over the top and a dash of The Zip [give generic name] for more color.

    1 head of cauliflower
    3 yellow crookneck squash
    4 zucchini
    2 yellow onions
    2 pkg. cherry tomatoes
    ½ celery root
    8 cloves garlic
    1 quart Fresh Silky Almond Milk
    1 container veggie broth
    Grapeseed oil

Preheat oven to broil. Cut the veggies into bite-size pieces. Place on non-stick cookie sheets and rub with grapeseed oil. Broil until lightly browned, 10-15 minutes. While veggies are roasting, make a almond milk and place in soup pot. When veggies are done, add cauliflower to the blender with half the onion and half the celery root and blend with enough of the almond milk to get a rich and creamy consistency. Place mixture in soup pot. Pulse chop the remaining veggies in a food processor until minced and add to soup. Stir to separate the bits. Add broth and stir well.

Scrap Soup. Serves 4
Donated by Mary Seibt

    3 large carrots
    2 celery stalks
    4 stalks asparagus

1 large yellow onion
6 cups of distilled water
4 tsps. of instant vegetable broth (yeast free)
1 1/2 tsps. cumin
2 tsps. dill
Real Salt to taste
2 tsps. 21 Spice Salute or Zip

Shred carrots and celery in food processor. Bring water to boil, adding vegetable broth and onion. Once boiling, turn off the heat. Add carrots, celery, stalks of asparagus and let stand until vegetables are tender. Cool enough to put in blender and mix all ingredients. Serve warm.

Veggie Almond Chowder. Serves 4
This soup is even better the next day after it has stored in the refrigerator overnight an the flavors have blended.

3 cups soaked almonds (blanch to remove skins if desired)
Juice of 1-2 lemons
1 garlic clove
1 tsp. Garlic Herb Bread Seasoning (Spice Hunter)
1 quart Veggie Broth (I use Pacific Brand)
2 tsp. dehydrated tomato powder (The Spice House)
1 tsp. real salt
½ tsp. cumin
½ tsp. celery salt
Black pepper or The Zip to taste (Spice Hunter)
¼ tsp. Green Thai Curry Paste
1 head broccoli
1 yellow onion
2-3 stalks celery
½ pound of fresh green peas from the pod

Put first 11 ingredients (up through curry paste) in a blender and blend until very smooth. Place in soup pot. Steam or steam fry the veggies, and add to soup pot. Warm and serve.

Tera's Any Meal Veggie Soup. Serves 6
Donated by Tera Prestwich

    1 Med. Onion
    3 Cloves of garlic (1tsp minced)
    5-7 Sun dried tomatoes
    2-3 Tbs. Bragg's liquid amino
    1 Tbs. parsley (1/4 c. fresh)
    2 tsp real salt
    Pepper to taste (I use 1 tsp)
    1 Quart Veggie broth
    1 Quart Water
    1 Head of cauliflower
    1 bunch of broccoli
    1 bunch of celery (I use the leaf also)
    1 lb of carrots
    ½ pd of fresh green beans
    ½ pd of peas

Blend first 7 ingredients (through pepper) in food processor. Put in Soup pot and cook until onion is clear. Add broth and Water and bring to a boil. Chop veggies (and feel free to get creative with any veggies here, instead of or in addition to the ingredients above), and add to the soup along with more water if necessary. Cook until veggies are just tender but still a little crunchy.

Celery Root Soup. Serves 4

Celery Root (or Celeriac) is different from celery, although the taste is a bit similar. Celery root is a large gnarly rough skinned root. Not the most attractive of vegetables sitting in the produce section, but none the less, delicious and very good for you. Wash celery root thoroughly with a brush to loosen dirt trapped in the gnarls. It is somewhat difficult to peel, so break out a good sharp knife or trusty peeler.

    Grapeseed oil
    1 large Celery Root, peeled and chopped into large bite-sized
    chunks
    2 white onions, chopped
    1 c. water or vegetable broth
    Real Salt to taste

Saute onions in oil until softened and lightly browned. Add celery root and water and steam for 5-10 minutes until veggies are done. Put soup in blender with enough water or broth to cover the top of the onion and celery root. Blend until smooth and creamy. Add more water if necessary to reach desired consistency, and season to taste with Real Salt. Serve warm as a soup, or spoon over veggies as a sauce or gravy. Experiment with adding your favorite seasonings.

Creamy Tomato Soup. Serves 2
Donated by Dr. Gladys Stenen

> 4 Roma Tomatoes
> 2 green onion tips (using about 1 inch of white/light green part)
> ¼ green pepper
> 1 cup vegetable broth
> 1 avocado or ¼ soft tofu package
> 1 tsp. sea salt
> pepper to taste

Liquefy in blender, then warm.

Creamy Curry Broccoli Soup. Serves 2
Donated by Dr. Gladys Stenen

> 2 cups of broccoli
> 2c. vegetable broth (adjust amount to reach desired thickness)
> ¼ soft tofu package (or more to taste)
> 1 tsp. curry powder
> Salt and Pepper to taste

Liquefy in blender, then warm.

Special Celery Soup*. Serves 6-8

This is a perfect soup for an appetizer before your main course, or on a day when you're tired and need to give your mind, body, and digestive tract, a rest.

> 1 Tbs. Coconut Oil
> 1 whole head of celery, including core and leaves, sliced
> 1 leek (sliced white part)
> 1 Tbs. ginger grated

1 quart Fresh Silky Almond Milk
Vegetable broth (optional)

Saute celery and leek [and ginger?] in oil until softened. Place half in the blender with half the almond milk and blend well. Mix with remaining veggies and almond milk and warm. Thin with vegetable broth if desired.

Green Gazpacho Two Ways. Serves 4-6
Donated by Eric Prouty

2nd place winner, the pH Miracle Recipe Contest

You can prepare this soup simply for a refreshing taste, or you can make it robust with the addition of herbs (which is what my family prefers). Either way, it's a wonderfully alkaline soup, packed with chlorophyll.

2 Avocados
2 Green Bell Peppers
6 Roma tomatoes
1-1/2 Large English Cucumbers (or 2 average size)
1 Head Romaine Lettuce
½ Red Onion
3 cloves Garlic
¼ cup fresh lemon juice
¼ t Real salt
2 Tbs. Olive oil
1-1/2 tsp. Basil
½ tsp. Dill
¼ tsp.Oregano
1/8 tsp. Sage powder

Chop all vegetables. Mix avocado, lemon juice and garlic in food processor (with S blade), until smooth and empty into bowl. Process tomatoes and romaine until smooth, and add to bowl. Pulse peppers, cucumbers and onion until chunky (approximately 1/8- ¼ inch) and empty into bowl. Mix well with salt and olive oil, and herbs if desired.

SALADS

Salad is a very important part of a meal, especially for someone with cancer. It is alkaline, high in water, and high in fiber, and should take up the major portion of your plate (70-80%).

Lentil-Brazil Nut Salad. Serves 1-2.
Donated by Roxy Boelz

3rd place, pH Miracle Recipe Contest

    1 ½ cups lentils, cooked
    1 cup edamame beans
    ¼ cup lime juice
    Dash of Real Salt
    ½ -1 tsp. fresh ginger
    1 cup spinach, rinsed and chopped
    2-3 Tbs. chopped Brazil nuts
    Sprinkle of parsley

Combine the lentils, edamame beans, and spinach. Combine the lime juice, salt and ginger, and stir into bean mixture. Sprinkle with brazil nuts and parsley.

Lemony Green Bean Salad, Serves 1-2
Donated by Roxy Boelz

3rd place, pH Miracle recipe contest

    1 cup green beans cut
    1 cup zucchini, sliced and cut
    juice of one lemon
    ½ cup daikon radish, sliced and cut
    ½ cup dulse flakes
    ½ cup parsley, cut

Lightly steam the green beans. Cool. Combine with zucchini and daikon. Stir in lemon juice. Sprinkle with dulse flakes and parsley.

Moroccan Mint Salad. Serves 4-6
Donated by Lisa El-Kerdi

Best in Show, pH Miracle Recipe Contest

Serve this refreshing salad with Lisa's other award winning recipe, North African Bean Stew!

   2 cucumbers, seeded and minced by hand
   4-6 scallions, minced by hand
   1 bunch parsley, stems removed
   1 bunch mint, stems removed
   ½-1 jalapeno
   4 tomatoes, seeded and finely chopped
   ½ cup lemon juice
   ¼ cup olive oil
   ½ tsp. Real salt
   ½ tsp. paprika

Mince herbs and jalapeno in food processor, or by hand. Mix in bowl with cucumbers and scallions. Add tomatoes, stir in lemon juice, olive oil and spices. Sahateck! (to your health)

Moroccan Cole Slaw. Serves 4-6
Donated by Eric Prouty

2nd place, pH Miracle Recipe Contest

   ½ Green Cabbage
   ½ Red Cabbage
   1/3 cup fresh Lemon juice
   1-1/2 tsp. Chinese 5 Spice powder
   ½ tsp. Caraway seeds
   4 Tbs. Olive Oil

Shred cabbage in food processor with shredder wheel. Mix all ingredients well in a bowl. Let sit for at least half an hour before serving to allow flavors to blend and seeds to soften.

More Peas Please
Donated by Dianne Ellsworth

This recipe would help to raise low blood sugar

    4 oz. Pea pods washed, trimmed and cut into bite sized pieces
    4 oz. Pea shoots 4 inches long cut in half (or pea sprouts 2 inches
    long)
    10 oz. Frozen baby peas thawed
    ½ of a small red onion sliced very thin cut slices in half
    2 cloves of garlic pressed through a garlic press or minced finely
    ¾ cup raw pumpkin seeds
    2 Tbs. fresh baby dill weed
    2 Tbs.. freshly grated ginger
    Zest of ½ lemon cut in ½ inch pieces
    Juice of 1 lemon
    3 Tbs. olive oil
    2 Tbs. grape seed oil
    1 Tbs. Udo's oil
    ½ tsp. dried dill weed
    ½ tsp. Spice Hunter Garlic Herb bread Seasoning
    Bragg's to taste

Mix the first 9 ingredients (through lemon zest) in a salad bowl. Make
a dressing by mixing the remaining ingredients together thoroughly.
Pour half of the dressing over the vegetable mixture and toss well.
Add more dressing to taste.

Alkalarian Cole Slaw. Serves 4-6
Donated by Sheila Mack

3rd place, The PH Miracle Recipe Contest

    ½ head green cabbage, shredded
    2 medium carrots, shredded
    ½ small red onion, sliced thinly into strips
    ½ cup chopped Italian parsley
    1 c coconut milk (make it fresh by blending the coconut water and
    meat of a Ti coconut) in a blender.
    1 t arrowroot powder (optional)
    ½ tsp. sea salt or to taste

¼ tsp. celery seed
½ Tbs. fresh lime juice
2 Tbs. Grapeseed Oil
Dash of cayenne pepper
Stevia (optional)

Toss the first four ingredients (through parsley) in a bowl. Blend coconut milk and arrowroot (if needed to thicken) in blender. Blend in remaining ingredients and toss with cabbage mixture. This tastes best if you let it sit and chill for awhile before serving, to give the flavors a chance to blend.

Popeye Salmon Salad. Serves 4
Donated by Maraline Krey

2nd place, pH Miracle Recipe Contest

This salad would also be delicious without the fish! To get the most juice out of them, roll the lemon and limes on the counter before cutting and squeezing them.

1 ½ lb. Salmon Fillet (cold water preferred)
juice of 1 lemon
juice of 3 limes, divided
4 oz. water
2 oz. Avocado Oil or Extra Virgin Olive Oil
Real Salt
Ground Pepper
1 oz. Ground flax Seed
1 oz. Poppy seed
handful of pine nuts (optional)
1 lb. Spinach leaves
½ cup of Basil leaves
1 cup Hearts of Palm, diced
1 cup diced carrots (optional)
1 cup diced celery (optional)
1 cup diced tomato (optional)
1 cup diced asparagus (optional)

Place salmon in a glass baking dish. Marinate in water and juice of lemon and one lime for two hours, turning over after an hour. Preheat oven to 400° F. Bake salmon in the liquid for 25 minutes, then place under the broiler for 5 minutes to brown the top. Make dressing by combining remaining lime juice, oil, pepper and salt, and seeds and pine nuts. Use kitchen scissors to cut spinach and basil leaves into bite-sized pieces. Add into a large salad bowl with whichever of the diced vegetables you choose. Toss with dressing and let sit until salmon is ready. To serve, cover dinner plates with salad, and top with pieces of salmon.

Rustic Guacamole makes an excellent accompaniment.

Quinoa Salad. Serves 4
Donated by Charlene Gamble

Quinoa is a versatile grain. Small and lacy, it makes a good substitute for rice. Because of its rice and beans, this recipe will help raise blood sugar levels.

½ cup Quinoa
1 cup vegetable broth
1 tsp. cumin, divided
½ cup brown rice
1 cup water
1 15 oz. Can black beans, drained, rinsed and drained again
1 ½ red peppers, finely diced
1/3 cup minced cilantro
1 ½ bunches green onion, chopped
2 celery sticks, chopped
4 Tbs. fresh lime juice
3 Tbs. Olive Oil (or whatever healthy oil you prefer)
VegeSal or Real Salt to taste

In a small saucepan, combine rice, water and half of cumin. Bring to a boil, cover, reduce heat and simmer 35 minutes. Rinse quinoa in sieve. In another small saucepan, combine with broth and half of cumin. Bring to a boil, cover, reduce heat and simmer 15-20 minutes. Combine [cooled?] grains in a bowl with remaining ingredients. Refrigerate for awhile before serving to blend flavors.

Tera's Hearty Party. Serves 4-6.
Recipe donated by Tera Prestwich

    1 head of Broccoli
    1 head of Cauliflower
    1 red bell pepper
    1 green bell pepper
    1 orange bell pepper
    2 stalks of celery (sliced)
    1 bag of edamame (soy beans)
    3 green onions
    ½ clove of minced garlic
    ¼ cup of Braggs Aminos or 1-2 tsp Real Salt
    ½ cup Essential Balance Oil (or oil of choice)
    1 Tbs. Garlic herb bread seasonings (Spice Hunter)
    Garnish with Zip (Spice Hunter)

Chop broccoli, cauliflower, celery, green onions and bell peppers and mix together. Cook Edamame's as directed and add to mix. Then add in the Essential Oil, minced garlic, Braggs Aminos, and Garlic Herb Bread Seasonings. Toss together and garnish with Zip.

Jerusalem Salad. Serves 4
Recipe donated by Sue Mount

    1/3 cup tahini
    2 Tbs. Olive Oil
    1-2 cloves garlic, crushed
    Juice of 1/2 lemon
    3 Tbs. parsley
    Salt/RealSalt to taste
    Water
    1 cucumber, diced
    6 roma tomatoes, or 3 regular tomatoes, diced

Mix first 6 ingredients thoroughly in a salad bowl; add water to thin to make a dressing. Add cucumber and tomatoes and toss. You can let this sit for an hour to allow the flavors to meld.

Refreshing Grapefruit Salad. Serves 2-4
Donated by Kathleen C. Waite

I like to arrange the avocado slices in this recipe like flower petals, and put the grapefruit mixture inside as the center of the flower. This recipe would help to raise low blood sugar.

1 Tbs. flax oil
1 Tbs. Braggs Liquid Aminos (or Real Salt or Herbamare to taste)
1-2 tsp. sesame seeds
1 tsp. Mexican Seasoning the Spice Hunter (optional)
1 grapefruit peeled and cut into bite size pieces
1 cup chopped celery
1 red bell pepper chopped or thinly sliced
1 cup jicama grated
1 handful of fresh cilantro
1 avocado peeled and sliced lengthwise
Soaked almonds, chopped

Combine first four ingredients (through mexican spice) to make dressing. Combine remaining ingredients except avocado and almonds in a bowl and toss with dressing. Arrange on a plate with avocado slices. Top with almonds.

Steamed Beets with Greens. Serves 2-4
Donated by Kathleen Waite

This recipe would be good to raise low blood sugar levels.

1 bunch of fresh beets with greens attached
½ juiced lemon
1 Tbs. flax oil
1 Tbs. Bragg Liquid Aminos (or Real Salt or Herbamare to taste)
Almonds, soaked and chopped (optional)

Cut beet head from greens and scrub well. Trim ends and cut into quarters or halves, depending on the size of the beet. Steam in steaming basket on high for 10 minutes and remove from heat. Meanwhile wash and rinse beet greens. Fold them over a couple of times and cut into pieces. When the beets are done, place the greens over the beets in the basket, put the lid back on, and let stand for 5 minutes to soften the greens. Meanwhile, combine lemon juice, oil and

Braggs or salt. Put greens and beets into a serving bowl and stir with dressing. Top with almonds.

Romaine Peppered Salad. Serves 6
Donated by Randy Wakefield

    1 clove minced or pressed garlic
    2 tsp. cold pressed olive oil or Esential Balance™
    2 tsp. minced onion
    2 tsp. tomato finely chopped
    1 sm. jalapeno pepper, seeded & finely chopped
    3 c. romaine lettuce
    3 c. Belgian endive
    1 red bell pepper, cut into strips
    1 yellow bell pepper, cut into strips
    Bragg's Amino's™/ Real salt to taste

Combine garlic and oil in a small bowl; let stand 30 minutes. Then add the minced onion, tomato, and jalapeno; stir well and set aside. Lay down whole romaine leaves to cover 6 salad plates. Tear endive and remaining romaine into small pieces and layer over top. Lay pepper strips on top. Drizzle each serving with 1 1/2 tablespoons of the oil mixture. Spray with Bragg's Amino's or Real Salt to taste.

DRESSINGS, DIPS AND SAUCES

The sauce is often the tastiest part of a meal. Veggies always taste more exciting dressed with herbs, seasonings and spices. It's also a way to include creamy textures in your dishes and enrich them with healthy and essential fats.

Almond Chili Sauce
Donated by Roxy Boelz

3rd place, pH Miracle Recipe Contest

Serves 2-4

    ½ cup raw almond butter
    1 Tbs. fresh ginger, grated
    2 Tbs. lemon juice

1 clove of garlic
1 Tbs. Bragg's Aminos
1 chili, such as Serrano
¼ cup water

Blend all ingredients together in blender till smooth. Add the water gradually, until you get the consistency you desire.

Mock Sour Cream
Donated by Roxy Boelz

3rd place, pH Miracle Recipe Contest

Serves 2-4

¾ cup coconut meat
1/3 cup brazil nuts (soaked overnight)
3 Tbs. olive oil
2 Tbs. lemon juice
1 Tbs. water
½ tsp. Real Salt

Blend all ingredients until smooth. Add water gradually to get the consistency you want.

Flaxseed Oil and Lemon Dressing
Donated by Roxy Boelz

3rd place, pH Miracle Recipe Contest held by the Innerlight Foundation, July 2003

Serves 2-4

½ cup lemon juice
¼ cup flaxseed oil or Udo's Blend
¼ cup water
1/3 bunch, fresh basil (or 1-2 tsp. dried)
2 cloves of garlic
¼ cup olive oil

Combine basil and garlic in blender. Add the rest of the ingredients and blend to desired consistency.

Sunnie Spread
Donated by Roxy Boelz

3rd place, the pH Miracle Recipe Contest

Serves 2-4

   1 cup sunflower seeds (soaked for 6 hours or overnight)
   1 cup almonds (soaked for 6 hours or overnight)
   2 Tbs. lemon juice
   ½ cup fresh herbs of choice (parsley, basil, cilantro ect.)
   1 Tbs. dulse flakes

Process sunflower seeds and almonds in food processor. Add remaining ingredients except dulse flakes and stir well. Sprinkle on the dulse flakes.

Variations: For garlic flavor, add chopped garlic to lemon juice and herbs, then combine with sunflower/almond mixture. Use 1 tsp. kelp instead of dulse flakes, adding kelp in the food processor with the rest of the ingredients.

Almond Butter Dressing
Donated by Debra Jenkins

1st place winner, Transitional Recipes, in the pH Miracle Recipe Contest

Serves 2-4

   1-2 Tbs. Almond Butter
   ¼ pound Soft or Silken Tofu
   1 fresh clove garlic
   2-4 Tbs. oil (Udo's blend, Essential Oil blend, or olive oil)
   Juice of 1 Lime
   ½-1 Tbs. Liquid Bragg's Amino's
   1 tsp. Spice Hunter Mesquite Seasoning
   ½ tsp. onion powder

Blend ingredients together.

Tofu Hummus
Donated by Debra Jenkins

1st place winner, Transitional Recipes, in the pH Miracle Recipe Contest

Serves 2-3

  8 oz Tofu
  ½ cup raw Tahini
  ½ lemon juiced
  1 tsp. cumin
  2-3 sun dried peppers or tomatoes
  1 clove garlic
  ½ tsp. Real Salt

Blend all ingredients together.

Almond Gravy
Donated by Debra Jenkins

1st place winner, Transitional Recipes, the pH Miracle Recipe Contest

Serves 2-3

This is good over buckwheat, rice, veggie burgers, vegetables, salmon and more.

  2 cups water
  ½ cup almonds (soaked and blanched, if preferred)
  2 Tbs. Arrowroot powder
  2 tsp. Onion powder
  2 Tbs. Grapeseed oil
  ½ tsp. Real salt

Blend ingredients together. Then warm over high heat, stirring constantly until thickened, about about 3 minutes.

Tofu "Whipped Cream"
Donated by Debra Jenkins

1st place winner, Transitional Recipes, in the pH Miracle Recipe Contest held by Innerlight Foundation

Serves 2-4

  [would you like to make some suggestions on how to use this?]

106

½ pound (8oz) Silken Tofu
2 tsp. Frontier non-alcoholic Vanilla
1/8 tsp. Stevia
1 Tbs. lemon juice
water or almond milk
1 ½ tsp. Psyllium or agar flakes (optional)

Drain tofu thoroughly. Combine tofu, vanilla, stevia and lemon juice in food processor and blend. Add water or almond milk as need to create a smooth consistency (should take only a few tablespoons). To make whipped cream stiffer, add psyllium or agar. Refrigerate until chilled.

Variation: flavor with cinnamon.

Nutty Cream Topping
Donated by Debra Jenkins

1st place winner of Best Transitional Recipes, in the pH Miracle Recipe Contest

Serves 1-2

½ cup almonds
1/3 cup boiling water
½ tsp. lemon juice
Stevia

In a blender or coffee grinder, grind almonds to a fine powder. Add water and juice, and stevia to taste (about 2-3 drops of liquid or one packet). Blend on high till smooth and creamy. Chill for an hour or two.

Variation: flavor with cinnamon, or almond or maple flavoring (be sure to get the flavors without alcohol)

Almond Avocado Dressing Serves 2-4
Donated by Debra Jenkins 1st place winner of Best Transitional recipes in the pH Miracle Recipe Contest

2 Tbs. raw almond butter
1 clove garlic
½ medium avocado

1 Tbs. fresh lemon juice
1 Tbs. Bragg's Aminos
3 Tbs. Essential Oil Blend
3 Tbs. Udo's Oil Blend (or favorite olive oil)
Dash of garlic powder
¼ tsp. onion powder
½ tsp. Frontier Spice Fajita Seasonings

Blend in blender until smooth and creamy. Chill.

Variation: Add 3-4 sun dried tomatoes

Avocado Grapefruit Dressing. Serves 1-2
Donated by Debra Jenkins 1st place winner for best transitional recipes, in the pH Miracle Recipe Contest

1 large avocado
½ large grapefruit
Stevia (optional)

Blend

Blend 1 large avocado with ½ large grapefruit. Add stevia to balance tang, if desired.

Red Pepper Jelly
Donated by Cheri Freeman 3rd place winner of Transitional recipes in the pH Miracle Recipe Contest,

Yield: 1 ½ c; Serves 4

This keeps a few days in the fridge, or you can freeze it to use later. For a great snack, make little triangle sandwiches with warm sprouted wheat tortillas cut into quarters, almond butter and red pepper jelly.

2 Red Bell Peppers
30 drops Stevia (or to taste)
½ c. + 3 Tbs. Water
4 tsp. Pomona's Universal Pectin
4 tsp. Calcium Water (packet comes with pectin)

Grind or puree peppers in blender or food processor with 3 Tbs. Water. Add stevia to taste. Pour into a bowl. Prepare calcium water, and stir into pepper mixture. Bring ½ c water just to a boil and pour into food processor or blender. Quickly add pectin and blend. (You must work fast, or the pectin will form globs.) Quickly pour pectin mixture into bowl with pepper mixture and stir well. Pour into glass jar and refrigerate. It will jell completely in a couple hours.

Chips and Salsa. Serves 4
Donated by KELLY ANCLIEN

1st place winner of BEST alkalizing recipes, in the pH Miracle Recipe Contest held by the Innerlight

This recipe is great served as part of Kelly's other recipe, Fiesta Tacos El Alkalarian.

Sprouted wheat tortillas
Olive oil
Garlic pepper
Fajita seasoning
Real salt
2 large tomatoes
5 Tbs. diced purple or red onion
1 ½ jalapeno pepper, seeded and chopped (mild salsa)
3 tsp. chopped fresh cilantro
2 garlic cloves minced
1 tsp. fresh lemon juice
Real Salt to taste
½ tsp pepper
2 sun dried tomatoes (optional)

Preheat oven to 350 degrees. Rub oil onto both sides of each tortilla, and sprinkle one side with spices (those above, or any combination you dream up). Use a pizza cutter to slice each tortilla into 8 triangles. Bake on a cookie sheet for 13 minutes, or until crispy. Meanwhile, make the salsa. Place the remaining ingredients into a food processor and blend to desired consistency. Use the sun dried tomatoes if desired to sweeten and thicken the salsa.

Decadent Dill Spread. Serves 4
Donated by Eric Prouty

2nd place winner for alkalizing recipes, in the pH Miracle Recipe Contest held by the InnerLight

Spread on cucumber slices, celery stalks, sushi nori paper (for veggie rolls), flax crackers, or sprouted tortillas (for veggie wraps)

> 2 cups soaked sunflower seeds
> 3 cloves garlic
> 1/3 onion
> 2 Tbs. Olive Oil
> 1 Tbs. Bragg's Liquid Aminos (or ½ to 1 tsp. Real Salt)
> 1 tsp. Dill

Use Green Star/Green Life or Champion Juicer with plug attachment for nut butters. Add seeds, garlic and then onion. Mix with other ingredients in a bowl.

Tomata Tostada Basilicious
Donated by Dianne Ellsworth

Use your favorite pre-made tortillas for this recipe. Or, make your own. Dianne likes to tweak the Super Tortillas recipe The pH Miracle by adding about 20 sun dried tomatoes, an additional 2-4 basil leaves, roasted green chili, a peeled and seeded, and reducing the amount of coconut milk or water to achieve the correct consistency for dough.

> 2-3 T olive oil
> juice of 1 lime
> 1-2 garlic cloves, minced
> 1/8-¼ c tahini (raw)
> 1 17 oz. jar garbanzo beans, drained (save water)
> 20-22 sun dried tomatoes packed in olive oil
> 8-10 basil leaves (plus additional for garnish)
> Real Salt, to taste
> ½-1 t Garlic Herb Bread Seasoning (Spice Hunter)
> ½-1 t cumin
> Zip (Spice Hunter), to taste
> Tortillas
> Tomatoes, sliced
> Guacamole

In a food processor put oil, lime juice, garlic, and tahini and process until smooth. Add beans, sun dried tomatoes and seasonings and process until creamy. You may need to thin with extra water (from beans) to desired consistency. Spread hummus on tortillas, add a layer of tomato slices and a layer of guacamole, and garnish with sliced basil leaves.

Texas Style Guacamole. Serves 2
Serve chilled or at room temperature, with veggies or tortilla chips (try the homemade tortilla chips with Mexican Seasoning in *The pH Miracle*). This is a great after work pick-me-up snack.

Donated by Amy Efeney

  2 large avocados
  1 whole jalapeno pepper (more or less)
  ½ habanero pepper (or not- they're really hot!)
  ¼ cup onion
  ¼ cup roasted tomatoes (or fresh)
  1 tsp. fresh lemon juice
  1 shot garlic powder
  1 shot Redmond Real salt
  1 or 2 shots fresh ground pepper

Mash all ingredients together with a fork for chunky guacamole, or use a blender (a new one might have a "salsa" setting) or food processor for smoother texture.

Avocado Salad Dressing. Serves 4-6
Donated by Gerry Johnson

Delicious over a garden salad.

  2 ripe avocados, peeled
  1 cup freshly juiced celery juice
  Seasonings (optional)

Mix together in a blender, adjusting amount of juice to achieve desired consistency. Add whatever seasonings appeal to you-or enjoy as is.

Sunshine Dressing. Serves 6-8
Donated by Frances Parkton

2nd place, in the pH Miracle Recipe Contest

This is a great versatile dressing, dip, or sauce. Somewhat like an all around Hollandaise Sauce that you could use for most any dish. Great over tacos or burritos too!

    2 cups minced cucumber
    2 sun-dried tomatoes
    1 cup onions minced
    4 jalapenos minced
    1 cup Green bell pepper minced
    ½ cup Olive oil
    ½ cup Avocado Oil
    ¼ cup. Veganaise (make sure it doesn't have vinegar)
    2 tsp. Mexican Seasoning
    Juice of 2 limes
    2 tsp. of Herbamare
    ½ tsp. cayenne pepper
    2 tsp. fresh garlic

Put all ingredients in vitamix or blender and blend to make salad dressing. Adjust seasonings to taste.

Variation: add 1 c- 4 pints cherry tomatoes for a wonderful gazpacho. Or serve over a bowl of the following combination: 2 c. cooked quinoa, 1 c. minced zucchini, 2 c. minced broccoli, 1 c. minced onion, 1 red or orange bell pepper, minced, 1 cup pine nuts, 2 T toasted sesame oil, and salt, tomatoes, and parsley to taste.

Rustic Guacamole. Serves 4-6
Donated by Maraline Krey

2nd place in transitional recipes, in the pH Miracle Recipe Contest held by the InnerLight Foundation

This rustic guacamole can be served as a side dish, as a main course salad over baby spinach drenched in lime juice and and avocado or olive oil. For a great salsa to use over fish, add a cut up grapefruit.

    4 Haas Avocados, diced into ½-3/4 inch cubes
    ½ bunch cilantro, cut up (use kitchen scissors)

1 x-large or 2-3 small tomatoes, diced
¼ onion, chopped
juice of 2 or 3 limes
½ tsp. Real Salt
½ -1 tsp. The Zip (Spice Hunter) or hot sauce (optional)

Combine in a large bowl and toss as you would a salad. Keeps in the refrigerator for two days.

Pesto Dressing/ Sauce. Serves 4

Serve cold over salad or veggies or legumes.

½ jar Garlic Galore Pesto (Rising Sun Farms brand, has no dairy)
½ cup Olive Oil (cold pressed virgin)
2-3 sundried tomatoes
1 tsp. Garlic Herb Bread Seasoning (Spice Hunter)
½ cup raw Macadamia Nuts
water to desired consistency

Put all ingredients into a food processor and process until smooth, adding water to desired consistency.

Fresh Garlic Herb Dressing. Serves 4

¾ C. Essential Balance Oil, a blend of organic flax, pumpkin and sunflower oils (Omega Nutrition)
Juice of one large lime
1 tsp. Italian Pizza Seasoning (Spice Hunter)
2-3 cloves fresh Garlic minced
½ tsp. Onion Salt (Real Salt puts out a nice blend)
½ tsp. vegetable Rub (Spice Hunter)
¼ tsp. fresh minced rosemary
¼ tsp. heat wave Seasoning (very hot spice) (The Cape Herb and Spice Company)

Blend all ingredients in a food processor or blender until well blended.

RANCHadamia Super Sauce. Serves 6-8

This is a great way to get off of dairy ranch salad dressing. It is also great as a dip for raw veggies, or as a spread in wraps. Macadamias are rich in unsaturated fats, and contain calcium, magnesium, and many of the amino acids that make complete proteins.

> 2 cups of fresh raw macadamia nuts
> Juice of 1 lemon
> 2-6 tsp. of LiteHouse Salad Herbs seasoning (a freeze-dried combination of parsley, shallots, chives, onions and garlic)
> 6-9 sundried tomatos
> 1 and 1/2 tsp. Spice Hunter Cafe Sole Lemon Pepper (a blend of lemon, pepper, onion, and sea salt)
> 2 squirts of Braggs Aminos
> water

With food processor running (using an S-blade), add all ingredients except water through the top shoot. Start with 2 t of seasoning, then taste and adjust the amount. Mix well and then slowly pour a large glass of water in until you reach desired consistency. Process until very creamy.

3 Citrus Dressing

About 2 c; Serves 6-8

This is a nice thick dressing with a sweet and our taste…very zingy! It is good when you are phasing out Thousand Island and other sweet dressings.

> juice of ½ large Pink Grapefruit
> juice of 1 lime
> juice of 1 lemon
> ½ tsp. Chickory root powder (name brand Nature's Taste by Amazon) OR 6-10 drops of liquid Stevia
> extract or 1 -2 packets of powdered Stevia.
> 1 tsp. hot mustard powder
> 4 Tbs. dried onion
> 2 tsp. garlic powder
> 2 tsp. dried basil
> ¼ tsp. dried rosemary
> ½ tsp. real salt
> pinch of Zip or to taste
> 1 ½ c Essential Balance Oil (Arrowhead Mills or Omega Nutrition

brand) or other healthy oil
1 heaping Tbs. flaxseeds

Put all but last 2 ingredients into a food processor [or blender?] and blend well. With machine still running, add oil, then flaxseeds, and let machine run until all ingredients are well emulsified.

Citrus Flax and Poppyseed Dressing. Serves 4
Recipe donated by Derry Bresee

½ cup carrot juice
½ cup freshly squeezed citrus juice (juice of 2 lemons, ½ grapefruit to =1/2 cup)
½ tsp. dry powdered mustard
2 Tbs. minced dry onion
1 t flaxseeds (optional)
1 tsp. minced fresh garlic
1 tsp. basil
½ tsp. Salt
1 T poppy seeds
1 c flaxseed oil

Combine all but the last two ingredients in a blender and blend, using the flaxseeds if you want a thicker dressing. Add poppy seeds and pulse briefly. With blender on low, slowly pour oil in until dressing is emulsified and thickened.

Flaxseed Oil Dressing. Serves 2-4
Recipe donated by Derry Bresee

Juice of 1 lemon or lime, about ¼ cup
½ tsp. onion powder
½ tsp. garlic powder
½ tsp. salt
½ tsp. chop dry basil
1 T flaxseeds (optional-use if you want to thicken enough that it spreads like mayonaise)
½ c Flaxseed oil (or, enough to be twice as much as the juice)
(Shake the bottle well before pouring)

Blend in blender. Serve immediately, or refrigerate until use.

Variation: use your favorite herbs or spices instead of the seasonings listed here.

ENTREES/SIDE DISHES

The following dishes range from casual to gourmet, and offer some of the best sources of animal protein, good fats, and complimentary seasonings. Whether they are entrees or side dishes depends on the balance you need to strike, keeping at least a 70/30 ratio on your plate, with the majority of your meal being raw veggies.

Coconut/Macadamia Nut Crusted Salmon. Serves 6

This is a wonderfully sweet Hawaiian rendition of salmon I use for special occasions. It always gets rave reviews at The pH Miracle retreats!

> 6 Salmon Filets sliced very thin (1/2 inch)
> 3 cups dehydrated unsweetened coconut flakes
> 3 cups raw macadamia Nuts
> 1 tsp. real salt
> 2 tsp. Garlic Herb Bread Seasoning
> 1 can coconut milk (Thai brand)
> Juice of three limes
> Grapeseed Oil for frying

Combine coconut, macadamias, salt and seasoning in food processor. Pulse chop to mix, then let the machine run until the mixture is finely ground and crumbly. Combine lime juice and coconut milk. Dip filets in the liquid, then into the coconut mixture to coat heavily. Press and pat the coating into the fish. In an electric frying pan on medium heat, fry 4-6 minutes, or until golden browned. Flip just once and fry on the other side until golden. If the fish is not done in the center, place the lid over the frying pan and steam until done. Lift each filet onto a serving platter with a spatula, taking care lest the coating from crumble off. Serve immediately.

Asparagus with Garlic-Lemon Sauce
Donated by Roxy Boelz

3rd place for alkalizing recipes, in The pH Miracle Recipe Contest held by the Innerlight Foundation, July

Serves 1-2

 2 cups of asparagus, steamed
 1/3 cup fresh lemon juice
 3 Tbs. ground golden flaxseed
 1 chopped garlic clove

Lightly steam asparagus. Add lemon juice, garlic and ground flaxseed and stir. Serve warm or cold.

Tomato Asparagus Ratatouille
Donated by Debra Jenkins

1st place in transitional recipes, in the pH Miracle Recipe Contest held by the Innerlight Foundation, July

Serves 2-4

Serve on its own, or over wild rice, buckwheat, or spelt noodles. Makes a great alkaline anytime meal… even breakfast!

 1 medium eggplant (peeled and cubed)
 1 cup chopped asparagus
 ½ cup chopped green beans
 1 chopped onion
 1 clove garlic (minced or grated)
 1 small zucchini (sliced)
 3-4 fresh tomatoes
 1-2 cups fresh spinach (optional)
 ¼ cup olive oil (can use Garlic flavored or Rosemary for extra flavor)
 ¼ tsp. Cayenne Pepper
 ½ tsp. garlic powder
 1 tsp. onion powder
 1-2 tsp. Spice Hunter Mesquite Seasoning
 Real Salt and or Bragg's Aminos to taste

Lightly "saute" all vegetables except spinach in water in a skillet for 2-4 minutes. Stir in seasonings. Add spinach (if using) and stir for 30 seconds more. Remove from heat, pour olive oil over all, and spray with Bragg's Aminos. Serve immediately.

Variation: add a few white beans or tofu

Fiesta Tacos El Alkalarian
Donated by Kelly Anclien

best Transitional recipe in recipe contest held by Innerlight Foundation July 2003

Serves 4-6

> 2 sprouted wheat tortillas
> olive oil
> Spice Hunter Garlic Pepper
> Fajita Seasoining
> Real Salt
> 2 large tomatoes peeled and seeded
> 5 Tbs. diced purple or red onion
> 2 sun dried tomatoes
> 1 ½ tsp jalapeno pepper, seeded (mild salsa)
> 3 tsp. fresh cilantro
> 2 garlic cloves minced
> 1 tsp. fresh lemon juice
> ½ tsp. ground pepper
> 2 avocados, mashed with a fork
> ½ tsp. Spice Hunter's Mesquite
> ½ tsp. Spice Hunter's Fajita
> ¼ tsp Real Salt
> refried beans
> red bell peppers sliced into strips
> mixed greens

Line bottom oven rack with tin foil. Preheat oven to 350 degrees. Rub olive oil onto both sides of tortilla, and sprinkle one side with garlic pepper, fajita seasoning and salt. Hang each tortilla over 2 bars of the upper oven rack, to form the shape of tacos. (Any dripping oil will land on the tin foil.) Bake for 13 minutes, or until crisp. Meanwhile, make the salsa by blending tomatoes, onion, jalapeno, cilantro, garlic, lemon juice, and ground pepper in food processor to desired consistency. Use sun dried tomatoes if you like a sweeter, thicker salsa. Add real salt to taste. Make guacamole by stirring together avocado with mesquite and fajita seasoning and real salt. Assemble fiesta tacos with layers of refriend beans, salsa, guacamole, red peppers and mixed greens.

Roasted Veggie Pizzas. Serves 8-10

I developed this recipe by basically unwrapping "The Super Wraps" (from *The pH Miracle*), roasting the veggies, and crisping the tortillas. These are by far the favorite dinner at pH Miracle retreats. Feel free to add to or change the veggies you use in any way that appeals to you. Eggplant, bok choy, celery, and snow peas, anyone?

3 red bell peppers
2-3 orange bell peppers
1-2 green bell pepper
2 sweet onions (I use yellow)
20-30 whole pieces (cloves) of garlic
4 yellow crook neck squash
3 zucchinis
1-2 heads of broccoli flowerets
heads of cauliflower
Avocados, sliced
Sprouted wheat tortillas
Hummus
Non-dairy pesto
Sundried tomato paste (store bought, or made by whirling sundried tomatoes in a food processor)
Pine nuts or slivered almonds (optional)

Preheat broiler. Cut the veggies, except avocado, into bite sized chunks. Place on cookie sheets and lightly sprinkle with grapeseed oil. Broil until lightly browned on the edges. Meanwhile, spread a thick layer of hummus and pesto on each tortilla. Top with generous amounts of roasted veggies, and top with avocado and some squirts of sundried tomato paste. Sprinkle with nuts if desired. Place under broiler until tortillas have crisped and veggies are sizzling hot, and serve immediately.

Wild Fajita Verde

Donated by Lory Fabbi

Serves 2-3

Serve with Ensalada Mexico (following).

½ red bell pepper sliced in ¼" wide long strips
½ green bell pepper sliced in ¼"wide long strips
½ small white or yellow onion thinly sliced
½ cup cooked Kashi pilaf (whole grains) or brown rice
2 Tbs. Roasted green chilies diced
15 fresh cilantro leaves, rolled between fingers to crush
½ avocado sliced
Salsa Verde-I use Herdez brand (No vinegar)
Dash of Braggs liquid aminos if desired
2-3 Sprouted wheat tortillas or fresh homemade spelt tortillas OR
use large lettuce leaf in place of tortillas

Saute peppers in a small non-stick pan wiped sparingly with oil, or grill on a Foreman type grill, 3-4 minutes until tender but still crunchy. Cook onion slices the same way until translucent. Warm tortilla in pan, remove and fill with peppers nad onions. Top with cilantro, lime juice, avocado, rice or Kashi, and salsa verde.

Ensalada Mexico

Donated by Lory Fabbi

Serves 2-3

The perfect compliment to Wild Fajita Verde. Or, to make it a main course on its own, serve with homemade tortilla chips and a dip made of refried beans, salsa, lime juice, and chopped onion, thinned slightly with water.

½ sliced red onion
1 chopped bell pepper
½ cup chopped jicama
2-3 radishes sliced
1 chopped ripe tomato
½ avocado chopped
½ cup black or kidney beans (optional)
Salsa

Mix all but the last ingredient together, and top with your favorite fresh salsa (no vinegar).

Variation: Mix 1-2 T Veganaise with salsa (to taste) in food processor or blender for a creamier dressing. Or, to boost the spiciness, add ¼ jalepeno, peeled, seeded and chopped. (Warning: Wash hands immediately after handling jalepeno to remove hot pepper oil, which can otherwise really sting.)

pH Pizza Delight
Donated by David Martini

Serves 1-2

So fast, tasty and alkaline, you can enjoy this anytime.

    1 Sprouted wheat tortilla (large burrito size)
    Hummus
    Bell Pepper in assorted colors
    Fresh cucumbers
    Fresh Spinach
    Tofu
    Sun dried tomatoes packed in olive oil
    Spice Hunter Seasoning of your choice

Spread the hummus evenly on the tortilla. Cut the toppings into slices. (Roll spinach leaves up.) Place veggies on the hummus in whatever design or pattern you like. Sprinkle with your favorite

Spice Hunter seasoning. Slice into wedges and enjoy!

China Moon Vegetable Pasta With Coconut Lotus Sauce. Serves 6-8
Donated by Lisa El-Kerdi

BEST IN SHOW recipe in The pH Miracle Recipe Contest

This colorful and flavorful dish is highly adaptable. Feel free to add vegetables of choice, modify according to season, and adjust quantities to suit the number of friends you are serving.

    1 large or 2 small spaghetti squash
    1 bunch scallions, cut in 2" diagonals
    1 carrot, thinly sliced

1-2 Cups Broccoli Florets
½ lb. Asparagus, cut in 2" diagonals
1 red bell pepper, sliced
2 yellow squash, sliced
1 zucchini, sliced
4-6 tiny bok choy, leaves separated, or ½ stalk large bok choy, sliced
½ lb. Snow peas
½ c coconut lotus sauce (recipe follows)
shredded unsweetened coconut
black sesame seeds

Cover lower oven rack with aluminum foil to catch any drippings. Preheat oven to 375-400 degrees. Make a one inch slit in top of spaghetti squash. Bake on upper oven rack for 30-40 minutes, until squash gives to gentle pressure but is not mushy. Bring water to a boil in bottom of large pot with steamer tray, then reduce to simmer. Place vegetables in steamer starting with scallions and carrots and continuing in order listed above. Cover and steam gently for 3-5 minutes, then turn off heat. The stored heat will continue to cook the vegetables. Be careful not to let them get overdone! Cut squash in half and scoop seeds out of center. Run fork lengthwise along the inside of the squash to form "spaghetti", and scoop gently onto plates or into shallow bowls. When veggies are done, remove steamer tray from pot. (Save broth for a soup base!) Return vegetables to pot and toss gently with desired amount of sauce, and spoon on top of squash. Garnish with coconut and sesame seeds.

Coconut Lotus Sauce

Besides making China Moon vegetable pasta, you can use this versatile sauce on a stir fry or as a dressing or dip.

2" piece of ginger root, peeled and sliced
2 large cloves garlic
½ tsp. crushed red pepper flakes (adjust to desired heat)
½ cup Bragg's Liquid Aminos (or more to taste)
2 Tbs. toasted Sesame Oil
2 T flaxseed oil
¼ cup water, carrot juice, or vegetable broth (optional)

Real Salt to taste
Unsweetened coconut milk (I prefer Thai Kitchen) to taste

Blend first three ingredients in food processor or Vita Mix. Add Bragg's and blend until smooth. Pour into jar, add oils and coconut milk, and water and shake. Thin with water, carrot juice or vegetable broth if desired. Store in refrigerator.

Variations: for Thai lotus sauce, add juice of one lime, 2 T fresh or 1 t dried lemongrass, 1 T fresh of ½ t dried basil and chopped fresh cilantro if desired.

For basic lotus sauce, omit coconut milk and increase flaxseed oil to ¼-1/3 c.

For lotus dressing, to ½ c basic lotus sauce add ¼ c lime juice, 1 ½ c flaxseed or untoasted sesame oil, ½ carrot (optional) and ½ sweet onion (optional), and blend until smooth.

For Indonesian Dipping Sauce, to ¾ c. basic lotus sauce add 1 c almond butter, ¼ t crushed red pepper (or to taste), and ½-1 c unsweetened coconut milk to reach desired consistency.

NORTH AFRICAN BEAN STEW. Serves 4-6
Donated by Lisa El-Kerdi

BEST IN SHOW in the pH Miracle Recipe Contest held by the InnerLight Foundation, July 2003.

This rich and exotic stew is sure to spice up any gathering. Serve with Moroccan Mint Salad (following). This recipe would be good to raise blood sugars.

> 1 ½ cups uncooked 7 bean and barley mix (or any mix of dried beans), soaked overnight, rinsed, and drained
> 1 bay leaf
> 1/8 tsp. cinnamon
> 4 cloves garlic
> 2 onions, quartered
> 4 carrots, cut into chunks
> 4 stalks celery, cut into chunks
> 1 large or 2 small eggplant

Real Salt
1 red bell pepper
1 yellow bell pepper
½ tsp. turmeric
1 tsp. coriander
1 tsp. cumin
½ tsp. cardamom
1/8 tsp. black pepper
1/8 tsp. cayenne
3-4 cloves garlic, pressed
2 or 3 yellow squash
2 or 3 zucchini
4 chopped tomatoes or 1 box Pomi chopped tomatoes
1 tsp. real salt
Olive Oil

Cover beans with 2 ½" water in large pot and add bay leaf and cinnamon. Bring to boil and skim off foam. Reduce to low heat and simmer, covered, for 30 minutes. Chop garlic, onions, carrots, and celery in food processor. Add to beans after 30 minutes cooking. Simmer until beans are cooked, 1-1 ½ hour. Cube and generously salt eggplant. Let sit ½-1 hour. Chop peppers. Rinse eggplant and squeeze out juices. While eggplant is salting, sauté spices in olive oil. Add to beans. Add eggplant and peppers. Simmer ½ hour. Cut squashes in half lengthwise and slice. Add to stew. Simmer 10 minutes. Add tomatoes and salt to stew. Simmer 10 minutes. Adjust salt to taste. Ladle into deep bowls and top each serving with 1 Tbs. Olive Oil (or to taste).

Spicy Kale Slaw. Serves 4
Donated by Deborah Johnson

2nd place for Alkalarian recipes, in The pH Miracle Recipe Contest, held by the InnerLight Foundation

  1 ripe avocado, seeded and peeled
  2 cups peeled cubed jicama
  Juice of 1 lime
  1 scoop soy sprouts powder
  1 Tablespoon UDO's Choice Oil
  ½-teaspoon Real Salt or to tastePlace all of the above in a food processor or Vita Mix and blend until smooth, stop machine.

While above ingredients are still in processing bowl, add the following in order given:

1 carrot, washed and cut into 1 inch pieces
3 kale spines, cut into 1-inch pieces
1-1½ jalapeno pepper, depending on how hot you like your food.
1 tomatillo, peeled and quartered
½ tsp. mustard seeds
3 kale leaves (remove spine and cut into 1-inch pieces, add with carrot layer)
tear leaf portion into large pieces.

Process, just until all ingredients are chopped to desired consistency. If using a processor pulse and scrape bowl. If using a Vita Mix use tamping tool, do not over process. This is a good lunch for one or a great side dish for two.

Fantastic Kale. Serves 4
Donated by Wendy J. Pauluk

Kale is a calcium rich chewy dark green leafy vegetable. It is good juiced or in the raw salad below.

1 bunch Kale
¼ cup Olive Oil
1 small Red Onion
1 Red Bell Pepper
Juice of 1 lemon
The Zip seasoning

Tear Kale into bite-sized pieces. Do not use center stem. Slice red onion and red bell pepper into thin strips and add to kale. Add olive oil and toss. (You may add more or less depending on size) refrigerate overnight in covered bowl. Add juice of 1 lemon and Zip seasoning to taste before serving.

Super Stuffed Tomatoes. Serves 2-4

Donated by Frances Fujii

This beautifully presented recipe would help raise blood sugar levels.

6 medium-sized tomatoes
1 cup (dry) black beans
2 pkg. firm tofu
2 lb. Swiss chard, coarsely chopped (may substitute kale, spinach, beet greens or other preferred leafy green vegetable)
2 cups (uncooked) wild rice (or use ½ brown and ½ wild rice)
4 cloves garlic diced
1 medium onion diced
Bragg's liquid Aminos
Vegetable seasoning salt (I like Herbamare)
Macadamia Oil
Udo's Choice Oil or Olive Oil

Soak black beans overnight. Put in medium sized pot, add 2" water, bring to a boil. Simmer of 1 hour or until tender. Can use whole or slightly mashed. Season with seasoning salt and set aside. Cook wild/brown rice, Set aside. Lightly sauté onions and garlic and Macadamiz Oil. Add greens and small amount of water and steam-fry until just tender, about 5 minutes. Season with bragg's Liquid Aminos and set aside. Lightly sauté tofu in same pan and add seasoning slat to taste. Scoop out tomatoes. Dice scooped out sections and set aside. Bake hollowed-out tomatoes at 300 for 5-10 minutes to warm. (Do not over-bake or the tomatoes will get too soft). On individual serving plates, create a bottom "ring" of wild rice, with a second ring of seasoned black beans on top of it. Place a hollowed tomato in the center of the double-decker ring. Sprinkle tofu cubes around on top of the beans/rice at the base of the tomato and stuff the tomato with greens (spill greens to overflow the top of the tomato if desired). Sprinkle the raw diced tomatoes on top of the greens, drizzle a little Udo's Choice or Olive oil and serve. Note: If you like garlic, you can mix in roasted garlic to the warm cooked brown rice before serving.

Robio's Burrito. Serves 1
Donated by Robio

This burrito would make a great meal anytime… even for breakfast. It would also help to raise low blood sugars. You can add or subtract and cut/slice/dice the items listed below to your own specifications. This recipe is so versatile, and you can add your own spin on it every time to make it delicious and entertaining.

1 sprouted wheat , spelt, or grain tortilla
organic refried beans
1 avocado
Herdez Salsa (hot, medium, or mild)
Lettuce
Tomato
Green Pepper
Jalepenos
Onions
California white Basmati Rice seasoned with Spanish spices
(optional)

Place the refried beans directly down the middle of the tortilla, then add the other toppings as you like. Fold like a taco or roll up like a burrito.

Energizer-Alkalizer Breakfast. Serves 2
Donated by Susan Lee Traft

This breakfast keeps you going strong and feeling awesome for several hours.

¼ cup chopped Red Pepper
¼ cup chopped Onion
1 clove of minced Garlic
About 2 cups of mixed veggies
(such as Swiss Chard, Broccoli, Green Beans, Pea Pods, Zucchini, few slices of carrot. etc.)
1 to 3 Tbs. of golden flax seeds (ground in coffee grinder.. tastes like bread crumbs)
1 Tbs. of Udo's choice Blend Oil
Bragg's Liquid Aminos to taste

Bring water to a simmer under steamer basket in pot. Add Red Pepper, Onion, Garlic and mixed veggies all at once into steamer basket and cover. Lightly steam (no more than 5 minutes). Immediately remove veggies from heat and put into salad bowl. Add Oil, ground Flax Seed and Braggs. Mix well.

Coconut Curry Salmon Chowder. Serves 4

This is a sweet rich dish that would help to raise blood sugar levels

1 lb. Fresh Salmon
1 tsp. Real Salt
1-2 tsp. Garlic Herb Bread Seasoning (Spice Hunter)
1 yellow onion
8 stalks celery
6 carrots
2 cans coconut milk (I use Thai brand)
½ tsp. Thai Green Curry Paste (I use Thai brand)
1-2 pkg. powdered Stevia (I use the Stevia with fiber) (if using straight Stevia, then use much less)
1 cup fresh coconut
½ tsp. vanilla (I use Frontier brand with no alcohol)
1 cup fresh peas from the pod (optional)
1 cup fresh Spinach (optional)

Sprinkle fish with some Real Salt and Garlic Herb Bread Seasoning and steam fry or use some grape seed oil and fry until cooked through but still moist. Cut into small bite size pieces and set aside. Cut the onion, carrots, and celery into bit size chunks, and put into a soup pot and steam until bright and chewy. (do not over cook). Add the coconut milk, green curry paste, vanilla, and stevia and stir to mix. Add Salmon. Take 1/3 of the whole ingredients and puree in blender and then return to the soup for a thick colorful base. Add fresh peas from the pod and/or fresh spinach towards the end if you like, and warm before serving.

Steamed Fish and Greens. Serves 4

1 lb. Fresh Salmon, Trout, or Red Snapper filet with skin on
1 Tbs. fresh ginger cut in thin slices or grated
1 cup yellow chives
½ cup green chives
½ cup cilantro
4 cups fresh Kale
2 Tbs. Braggs Aminos
½-1 cup fresh coconut water (sweet) taken from a fresh coconut (I use a clean screwdriver and a hammer to make two holes into the top of a coconut and pour the water out into a measuring cup. Then I break open the coconut with the hammer and a sharp meat cleaver to get to the fresh coconut meat.)
Real Salt to taste

In a non stick fry pan lay fish, skin side down, and steam fry with the lid on until the fish is cooked through but also moist. Half way through, take the lid off and sprinkle the fish with Real Salt and Garlic Herb Bread Seasoning (Spice Hunter). When the fish is done, take out on a plate and set aside. Take the skin off the fish but leave any oils from the fish in the pan. Place the thinly sliced ginger in the oiled pan and cook until the ginger is browned. Add all other ingredients except cilantro and steam in the pan with the lid on until bright green and softened. Add the fish and the cilantro back in and steam one or two more minutes before serving.

Veggie Tofu Loaf. Serves 6

This is wonderfully colorful and nutritious way to enjoy Tofu at any meal or even snack time. It's great steaming hot from the oven or sliced cold or broken up over a salad. Use the firmest Tofu type for best holding results. I use Nigari brand Extra Firm. For a binder, I use Mauk Family Farms Wheat Free Crusts, a blend of gold and brown flax seeds, sesame seeds and sunflower seeds, with garlic, onion, celery seed, red bell pepper, parsley, sea salt and pepper, dehydrated at 105 degrees, and process them in my food processor until they are a powder consistency. The flax, sunflower, and sesame seeds add extra flavor and healthy fats.

1 lb. Firm or Extra Firm Tofu

129

½ to 1 tsp. Real salt (or to taste)
5 tsp. Mexican Seasonings (Spice Hunter)
2 tsp. Vegetable Rub (Spice Hunter)
4 tsp. Sun Dried Tomatoes minced (Melissa Brand packed in Olive Oil)
½ Red Bell Pepper diced
2 Tbs. diced celery
2 Tbs. diced soaked almonds
2 Tbs. Raw Wheat Free Crusts, ground to powder (Mauk Family Farms)

Use the food processor to dice all ingredients that need dicing. Then place all ingredients in food processor and pulse chop until well mixed. Place on a grape seed oiled pan and mold into a loaf or two smaller loafs, about 2 inches in height. Brush some Grape seed oil over the top of the loaf and sprinkle The Zip over the top. Bake at 400 for 20-30 minutes or until lightly browned on top. Serve warm or let it chill over night. Slice and serve cold.

Variation 1: **Garlic Veggie Tofu Loaf**.

1 lb. Extra Firm Nigari Tofu
½ tsp. to 1 tsp. Real Salt
2-4 roasted cloves of garlic
2 Tbs. Dehydrated Veggie Granules [is that the generic name you would use?]
4 tsp. diced celery
4 tsp. diced red bell pepper
2 Tbs. ground Raw Wheat Free Crusts

Sprinkle Garlic Herb Bread Seasoning over the top

Variation 2: **Buckwheat Veggie Tofu Loaf**

The binder for this variation is raw buckwheat flour. Grind raw buckwheat in your blender or grinder to make this flour fresh

1 lb. Extra firm Tofu
6 tsp. Veggie seasoning (spice Hunter)
6 tsp diced celery
3 tsp red bell pepper
3 tsp. diced sun dried tomato
5 tsp.Garlic Herb bread seasoning

½ to 1 tsp. real salt

3 tsp raw Buckwheat ground to flour

Top the loaf with 2 tsp. ground Raw wheat free crusts (reference above).

Variation 3: Basil Veggie Tofu Loaf

1 lb. Extra Firm Nigari Tofu

½ to 1 tsp. Real Salt

4 tsp. diced celery

4 tsp.diced red bell pepper

2 Tbs. vegetable seasonings (Spice Hunter)

4 tsp. ground flax seeds

4 tsp. ground soaked almonds

6-8 tsp. fresh diced Basil

Sprinkle Garlic Herb Bread Seasoning on Top.

Variation 4: Quinoa Veggie Tofu Loaf

1 lb. Extra firm Nigari Tofu

1 Tbs. of Pesto Seasoning (Spice Hunter)

2 Tbs. diced celery

2 Tbs. diced red bell pepper

4 tsp. minced sun dried tomato (packed in Olive Oil)

1 heaping Tbs. of Quinoa ground flour (grind in your blender)

Oil and place dehydrated veggie granules on top (the Spice House)

Can't Get Enough Eggplant. Serves 1-2
Recipe donated by Myra Marvez

1 eggplant

olive oil

celtic salt

Finely chopped onion, size chosen according to taste and size of eggplant(s).

Roast eggplant on open fire till it is mostly cooked. Cool and Peel all burned skin off. Chop eggplant into small pieces. Finely mince the onion. Place eggplant in bowl, add onion, olive oil, salt, and mix well.

Cherry Tomatoes AvoRado Style. Serves 2-4

This is a great appetizer or hors d'oeuvre, or it could be served as a salad course.

1 pint cherry tomatoes
Juice from 1/2 lime
1 Avocado
!/2 tsp. dried onion
1 Tbs. minced cilantro
1/8 tsp. Zip seasoning (Spice Hunter) (use more if you like extra spicy)
1/8 tsp. Real Salt
dehydrated vegetable granules (Make your own or buy them)

Slice tomato tops off and use a melon ball spoon to scoop out seeds and pulp of tomatoes. Drain on paper towels upside down. In food processor with an S blade add remaining ingredients and pulse chop into a well mixed chunky consistency. Fill tomato shells with mixture and sprinkle dehydrated veggie granules on top. Serve chilled.

Doc Broc Stalks-Coyote Style

The good news is that when Dr. Young first tried this dish, he thought he was eating fried potatoes! I love it when I can fake him out! The even better news is that this taste treat is actually made of broccoli. Even my 15 year old Alex (our perpetual transitional boy) always asks for seconds and thirds of these.

6 long broccoli stalks peeled and sliced thin about 1/8 of an inch.
1 yellow onion sliced thin and chopped
2 Tbs. grapeseed oil
½ to 1 cup Creamy Tomato Soup (see recipe below)
1-2 tsp. Garlic Herb Bread Seasoning (Spice Hunter)
1-2 tsp. Seafood Grill & Broil Seasoning (Spice Hunter)
1-2 tsp. Mesquite Seasoning (Spice Hunter)
½ tsp. ground yellow mustard
1-3 tsp. Soy Parmesan (alternative) cheese (dairy free) I use Soymage Vegan Parmesan

Place sliced onion and sliced broccoli stalks pieces in a non stick fry pan together and steam fry for few minutes until onions and broccoli heat up and steam so they slip and slide around the pan. Add the Grape seed oil and stir veggies on high heat while they brown and become somewhat roasted. Once they are evenly fry roasted, turn down the heat to low and add ½ cup of the creamy tomato Soup (more or less depending on how much sauce you want in with your stalks, you can always add the other ½ later). Then sprinkle in seasonings to coat the stalks and onions. Stir well to distribute all the seasonings evenly. Last sprinkle in the amount of desired Soy Parmesean and stir once more to mix well.

Creamy Tomato Soup. Serves 2
Donated by Gladys Stenen

4 Roma Tomatoes (or equivalent)
2 green onion tips (about 1 inch of white/light green part)
¼ green pepper
1 cup vegetable broth
1 avocado or ¼ soft tofu package
1 tsp. sea salt
pepper to taste

Liqefy in blender. Heat just to warm.

Doc Broc Brunch. Serves 6

This is a hearty Deep Green dish that has plenty of crunch with the broccoli stalks and soaked almonds added. Perfect for a brunch or side dish.

1 yellow onion
2 cloves fresh garlic
3 large heads of Broccoli
1 lb. of young green string beans
1 small bowl of soaked almonds
Grapeseed or Olive Oil
Real Salt to taste

Trim and peel Broccoli stalks. Then cut Broccoli into bite size pieces. Trim and break green beans into bite size pieces. Lightly steam Broccoli and Green Beans unit bright green. In a food processor, pulse chop the onion and garlic until fine, set aside. Put soaked almonds into the food processor with an S blade and pulse chop into almond slivers. In an Electric Fry Pan, Place oil and add onion/garlic mixture and sauté for a few minutes. Add steamed Broccoli/green beans and stir fry to mix in with the onions and garlic. Add slivered soaked almonds and continue to mix well. Put lid on electric fry pan and continue to steam for a few minutes longer if softer veggies are desired. Add real Salt to taste.

Doc Broc Casserole. Serves 4-6

1 pkg. Smart Ground by LiteLife (soy protein substitute)
Florets from 2 large bunches of Broccoli (save leaves and stocks out, peel and clean stocks)
1 small bunch of fresh Basil or Tarragon stemmed and minced
1 cup soft Tofu
1 tsp. ground mustard seed
2/3 cup Olive Oil
1-2 cups roasted or soaked and re-dehydrated almonds for topping
Real Salt and Spice Hunter's The Zip to taste.

Steam Broccoli with a little water in a covered pan for about 4-5 minutes until Broccoli is bright green and just crisp/tender. In a food processor, process the broccoli leaves and stocks until very fine(scrape down sides if necessary). Then add the soft Tofu, mustard, basil, into the food processor with the fine broccoli mixture and process. With the processor running, slowly add the Olive Oil until mixture is well emulsified and creamy. In a large Electric Fry Pan, heat a small amount of Oil and add the Soy Smart Ground, crumble it up and fry it for a couple of minutes, then add the steamed broccoli and pour the creamy sauce from the processor over the top and stir in well. Use roasted slivered or dehydrated almonds and cut them up into small bits in the food processor for extra crunch...Then sprinkle over the top of the broccoli mixture and serve. Or return the lid to the fry pan and steam the mixture a bit to soften the almonds and broccoli more. Add Real Salt and The Zip to taste.

Mary Jane's Super Simple Spaghetti. Serves 2.
Donated by Mary Jane Medlock

    1 medium spaghetti squash
    2 medium ripe vine tomatoes chopped
    Juice of one small lemon
    1-2 cloves of fresh garlic minced or chopped
    2-3 Tbs. of olive oil
    Fresh ground pepper
    1/4 teaspoon of oregano

Cut spaghetti squash in half (clean out seeds). In a baking dish put spaghetti squash (facing down) in a 375 degree oven. Bake for approximately 45 minutes or until done. Let cool for about 5 minutes. Using fork, scoop out the spaghetti squash into a bowl. Add the remaining ingredients and toss. Eat warm or cold.

ALKALINE FOODS CHART

Food Category	Food	Rating <-- highly acidic -- highly alkaline -->					
Breads	Corn Tortillas		x				
Breads	Rye bread			x			
Breads	Sourdough bread		x				
Breads	White biscuit			x			
Breads	White bread		x				
Breads	Whole-grain bread			x			
Breads	Whole-meal bread			x			
Condiments	Ketchup		x				
Condiments	Mayonnaise		x				
Condiments	Miso		x				
Condiments	Mustard		x				
Condiments	Soy sauce		x				
Dairy	Buttermilk		x				
Dairy	Cheese (all varieties, from all milks)		x				
Dairy	Cream		x				
Dairy	Egg whites		x				
Dairy	Eggs (whole)		x				
Dairy	Homogenized milk		x				
Dairy	Milk (not pasteurized)			x			
Dairy	Milk (pasteurized)		x				
Dairy	Yoghurt (sweetened)		x				
Dairy	Yoghurt (unsweetened)			x			
Beverages & Drinks	Beer	x					
Beverages & Drinks	Coffee	x					
Beverages & Drinks	Coffee substitue drinks		x				
Beverages & Drinks	Fruit juice (natural)		x				
Beverages &	Fruit juice (sweetened)	x					

Category	Item					
Drinks						
Beverages & Drinks	Liquor	x				
Beverages & Drinks	Soda/Pop		x			
Beverages & Drinks	Tea (black)	x				
Beverages & Drinks	Tea (herbal, green)			x		
Beverages & Drinks	Water (Fiji, Hawaiian, Evian)				x	
Beverages & Drinks	Water (sparkling)		x			
Beverages & Drinks	Water (spring)			x		
Beverages & Drinks	Wine		x			
Fats & Oils	Borage oil				x	
Fats & Oils	Butter		x			
Fats & Oils	Coconut Oil (raw)				x	
Fats & Oils	Cod liver oil			x		
Fats & Oils	Corn oil		x			
Fats & Oils	Evening Primrose oil				x	
Fats & Oils	Flax seed oil				x	
Fats & Oils	Margarine		x			
Fats & Oils	Marine lipids				x	
Fats & Oils	Olive Oil				x	
Fats & Oils	Sesame oil				x	
Fats & Oils	Sunflower oil			x		
Fruits	Acai Berry			x		
Fruits	Apples			x		
Fruits	Apricots			x		
Fruits	Apricots (dried)			x		
Fruits	Avocado (protein)					x
Fruits	Banana (ripe)		x			
Fruits	Banana (unripe)			x		
Fruits	Black currant			x		
Fruits	Blackberries			x		
Fruits	Blueberry			x		

Fruits	Cantaloupe			x		
Fruits	Cherry, sour				x	
Fruits	Cherry, sweet			x		
Fruits	Clementines			x		
Fruits	Coconut, fresh				x	
Fruits	Cranberry			x		
Fruits	Currant			x		
Fruits	Dates			x		
Fruits	Dates (dried)			x		
Fruits	Fig juice powder			x		
Fruits	Figs (dried)			x		
Fruits	Figs (raw)			x		
Fruits	Fresh lemon				x	
Fruits	Goji berries			x		
Fruits	Gooseberry, ripe			x		
Fruits	Grapefruit				x	
Fruits	Grapes (ripe)			x		
Fruits	Italian plum			x		
Fruits	Limes				x	
Fruits	Mandarin orange		x			
Fruits	Mango			x		
Fruits	Nectarine			x		
Fruits	Orange			x		
Fruits	Papaya			x		
Fruits	Peach			x		
Fruits	Pear			x		
Fruits	Pineapple		x			
Fruits	Pomegranate			x		
Fruits	Rasberry		x			
Fruits	Red currant			x		
Fruits	Rose hips		x			
Fruits	Strawberries			x		
Fruits	Strawberry			x		
Fruits	Tangerine			x		
Fruits	Tomato					x
Fruits	Watermelon			x		
Fruits	Yellow plum			x		

Category	Food	1	2	3	4	5	6
Grains & Legumes	Basmati rice			X			
Grains & Legumes	Brown rice		X				
Grains & Legumes	Buckwheat				X		
Grains & Legumes	Bulgar wheat			X			
Grains & Legumes	Couscous			X			
Grains & Legumes	Granulated soy *(cooked, ground)*				X		
Grains & Legumes	kamut			X			
Grains & Legumes	Lentils			X			
Grains & Legumes	Lima beans				X		
Grains & Legumes	Oats			X			
Grains & Legumes	Rye bread			X			
Grains & Legumes	Soy flour				X		
Grains & Legumes	Soy lecithin, pure						X
Grains & Legumes	Soy nuts *(soaked soy beans, then dried)*						X
Grains & Legumes	Soybeans, fresh				X		
Grains & Legumes	Spelt				X		
Grains & Legumes	Tofu			X			
Grains & Legumes	Wheat		X				
Grains & Legumes	white (navy) beans				X		
Meat, Poultry & Fish	Beef	X					
Meat, Poultry & Fish	Buffalo		X				
Meat, Poultry & Fish	Chicken		X				
Meat, Poultry & Fish	Duck		X				
Meat, Poultry & Fish	Fresh water fish		X				
Meat, Poultry & Fish	Liver			X			
Meat, Poultry & Fish	Ocean fish		X				
Meat, Poultry & Fish	Organ meats			X			
Meat, Poultry & Fish	Oysters			X			
Meat, Poultry & Fish	Pork	X					

Category	Food						
Meat, Poultry & Fish	sardines (canned)	x					
Meat, Poultry & Fish	Tuna (canned)	x					
Meat, Poultry & Fish	Veal	x					
Misc	Bee pollen				x		
Misc	Canned foods		x				
Misc	cereals (like Kelloggs etc)		x				
Misc	Hummus			x			
Misc	Rice milk			x			
Misc	Royal Jelly				x		
Misc	Soy Protein Powder			x			
Misc	Tempeh			x			
Misc	Whey protein powder			x			
Nuts	Almond				x		
Nuts	Almond butter (raw)				x		
Nuts	Brazil nuts			x			
Nuts	Cashews			x			
Nuts	Filberts			x			
Nuts	Hazelnut			x			
Nuts	Macadamia nuts (raw)			x			
Nuts	Peanut butter (raw, organic)		x				
Nuts	Peanuts		x				
Nuts	pine nuts (raw)				x		
Nuts	Pistachios		x				
Nuts	Walnuts			x			
Roots	Carrot				x		
Roots	Fresh red beet				x		
Roots	Kohlrabi				x		
Roots	Potatoes				x		
Roots	Red radish					x	
Roots	Rutabaga				x		
Roots	Summer black radish						x
Roots	sweet potatoes			x			
Roots	Turnip				x		
Roots	White radish (spring)				x		
Roots	Yams				x		

Category	Item					
Seeds	Barley			x		
Seeds	Caraway seeds				x	
Seeds	Cumin seeds				x	
Seeds	Fennel seeds				x	
Seeds	Flax seeds			x		
Seeds	Pumpkin seeds			x		
Seeds	Sesame seeds			x		
Seeds	Sunflower seeds			x		
Seeds	Wheat Kernel		x			
Sweets & Sweeteners	Agave nectar			x		
Sweets & Sweeteners	Alcohol sugars (xylitol and the other sacharides.		x			
Sweets & Sweeteners	Artificial sweeteners	x				
Sweets & Sweeteners	Barley malt syrup			x		
Sweets & Sweeteners	Beet sugar		x			
Sweets & Sweeteners	Brown rice syrup			x		
Sweets & Sweeteners	Chocolates		x			
Sweets & Sweeteners	Dr. Bronner's barley malt sweetener			x		
Sweets & Sweeteners	Dried sugar cane juice			x		
Sweets & Sweeteners	Fructose		x			
Sweets & Sweeteners	Halva [ground sesame seed sweet]		x			
Sweets & Sweeteners	Honey		x			
Sweets & Sweeteners	Maple Syrup			x		
Sweets & Sweeteners	Molasses		x			
Sweets & Sweeteners	Sugar (white)	x				
Sweets &	Sugarcane		x			

Category	Item					
Sweeteners						
Sweets & Sweeteners	Turbinado sugar		X			
Vegetables	Alfalfa				X	
Vegetables	Alfalfa grass					X
Vegetables	Artichokes				X	
Vegetables	Asparagus				X	
Vegetables	Aubergine/Egg plant			X		
Vegetables	Barley grass					X
Vegetables	Basil				X	
Vegetables	Bell peppers/capsicums (all colors)			X		
Vegetables	Blue-Green Algae		X			
Vegetables	Bok Choy			X		
Vegetables	Brussels sprouts				X	
Vegetables	Cabbage lettuce, fresh				X	
Vegetables	Canned vegetables	X				
Vegetables	Cauliflower			X		
Vegetables	Cayenne pepper				X	
Vegetables	Celery				X	
Vegetables	Chives			X		
Vegetables	Cilantro				X	
Vegetables	Comfrey			X		
Vegetables	Cooked vegetables (all kinds)		X			
Vegetables	Cucumber, fresh					X
Vegetables	Dandelion					X
Vegetables	Dog grass					X
Vegetables	Endive, fresh				X	
Vegetables	French cut (*green*) beans				X	
Vegetables	Frozen vegetables	X				
Vegetables	Garlic				X	
Vegetables	Ginger				X	
Vegetables	Ginseng			X		
Vegetables	Green cabbage, *(December Harvest)*			X		
Vegetables	Green cabbage, *(March Harvest)*			X		
Vegetables	Horse radish			X		
Vegetables	Jicama					X
Vegetables	Kale					X

		1	2	3	4	5
Vegetables	Kamut grass					X
Vegetables	Lamb's lettuce			X		
Vegetables	Leeks (bulbs)			X		
Vegetables	Lettuce			X		
Vegetables	Mushrooms		X			
Vegetables	Mustard greens			X		
Vegetables	Onion			X		
Vegetables	Oregano				X	
Vegetables	Parsnips			X		
Vegetables	Peas, fresh			X		
Vegetables	Peas, ripe			X		
Vegetables	Peppers			X		
Vegetables	Pickled vegetables	X				
Vegetables	Pumpkins (raw)			X		
Vegetables	Raw onions				X	
Vegetables	Red cabbage			X		
Vegetables	Rhubarb stalks			X		
Vegetables	Savoy Cabbage			X		
Vegetables	Sea Vegetables			X		
Vegetables	Seaweed (dulse, kelp, laver, etc)			X		
Vegetables	Shave grass					X
Vegetables	Sorrel				X	
Vegetables	Sourkraut		X			
Vegetables	Soy Sprouts					X
Vegetables	Spinach *(March harvest)*			X		
Vegetables	Spinach *(other than March)*				X	
Vegetables	Sprouted seeds (all kinds)					X
Vegetables	Squash (all kinds, raw)			X		
Vegetables	Straw grass					X
Vegetables	Thyme			X		
Vegetables	Tomatoes (raw)				X	
Vegetables	Tomatoes (sundried)			X		
Vegetables	Watercress				X	
Vegetables	Wheat grass					X
Vegetables	White cabbage			X		
Vegetables	Yeast		X			
Vegetables	Zucchini			X		

EXERCISE DAILY

"The Doctor of the Future will give no medicine, but will involve the patient in the proper use of food, fresh air, and exercise."
Thomas Edison

"We know that exercise is chemotherapy without side effects."
Dr Finn Scott Andersen MD.

Exercise for the Body, Mind and Spirit

The human race has been and in some cases is asleep, and has dreamed that money and property are the true wealth. The result from the years of focusing on temporal wealth is seen in the uneasiness that prevails everywhere and the increase in obesity, diabetes, and cancer. The good news is humanity is beginning to wake up. It is unfortunate that it takes human tragedy to realize that it is me, my spouse, my children, my extended families and my friends, that are the most important and most precious thing on planet earth. And the quality of life is determined foundationally by the quality of your health and those who you love and care for.

The statement that the people who make up a nation or a race are imperfect is no more true than a pile of lumber is imperfect. It is the carpenters business to take the lumber which is perfect and build a beautiful house. So it is with the spiritual man, to take the perfect materials that are everywhere in this present world and build by the perfect law of chemistry and biology, a perfected, harmonious human being. And with this material, apply the same laws to build a perfect society.

I perceive from my blood research that the blood is the basic material of which the human body is continually being created or formed. As is the blood, so is the body. Why? Because, body cells that make up muscle, bone, tissue and organs are created out of the red blood cell. The current idea that a body builder builds muscle with protein is a scientific illusion. The "New Biology" teaches that strong and lasting

144

muscles are built with blood not protein drinks and the quality and strength of the blood is determined by how much green food you eat and drink. How does one of the strongest mammals, the Silver Back Gorilla, build his large and strong muscles or the horse, elephant, cow and black and brown bear for that matter? Is it from drinking protein drinks or taking steroids? No! They all build their muscle with their blood which is built on a diet that is high in green plant foods!

Continuing with this thought, I also perceive, so is the body, so is the brain. And, as is the brain, so is the quality of thought. As a man or woman buildeth with green foods, so is he or she. And as a man or woman IS, so thinks he or she.

Solomon's temple is an allegory of a man or woman's temple -- the human body. This house is built without a sound of a saw or hammer. And the quality of that temple is dependent upon the quality of the green food, drink, and thought one puts into it. The saying "you are what you eat" or "you are what you think" is at the foundation of your "House of Health."

Your bodies are the temple of the living God. But man, blinded by selfishness and pride, searches here and there. Scours the heavens with his telescope, digs deep into the earth, and dives into the ocean's depths, in a vain search for the "Elixir of Life" that may be found between the soles of his feet and the crown of his head. Our human body is a miracle of organization. No work of man can compare with it in accuracy of its process and the simplicity of its law. This law is the law of the universe, the law of opposites or opposition.

As I perceive the complexity of the human body I realize this: at maturity, the human skeleton contains about 165 bones, so delicately and perfectly adjusted. The muscles are about 500 in number. The length of the alimentary canal is 32 feet. The amount of blood in an average adult is 5 liters weighing over 30 pounds or one-fifth of the total body weight. The heart is six inches in length and four inches in diameter, and beats seventy times per minute, 4200 times per hour, 100,800 per day and 36,720,000 per year. At each beat, two and one-half ounces of blood are thrown out of it, 175 ounces per minute, 656 pounds per hour, or about 8 tons per day.

All the blood in the body passes through the heart every three minutes. And during seventy years it lifts 270,000,000 tons of blood.

The lungs contain about one gallon of air at their usual degree of inflation. We breath, on an average, 1200 breaths per hour and inhale 600 gallons of air, or 24,000 gallons daily.

The aggregate surface of air-cells of the lungs, exceed 20,000 square inches, an area nearly equal to that of a room twelve feet square. The average weight of the brain of an adult is three pounds, eight ounces. The average female brain is two pounds, four ounces. The convolutions of a woman's brain cells and tissues are finer and more delicate in fiber and mechanism, which evidently accounts for the intuition of women. It would appear that the difference in the convolutions and fineness of tissue in the brain matter is responsible for the degrees of consciousness called reason and intuition.

The nerves are all connected with the brain directly, or by the spinal marrow, but nerves receive their sustenance and regeneration from the blood, and their motive power from the solar plexus dynamic. The nerves, together with the branches and minute ramifications, probably exceed ten million in numbers.

The skin is composed of three layers, and varies from one-eight to one-quarter of an inch in thickness. The average area of skin is estimated to be about 2,000 square inches. The atmospheric pressure, being fourteen pounds to the square inch, a person of medium size is subject to a pressure of 40,000 pounds. Each square inch of skin contains 3,500 sweat tubes, or perspiratory pores (each of which may be likened to a little drain tile) one-fourth of an inch in length, making an aggregate length of the entire surface of the body 201,166 feet, or a tube for draining the body of endogenous acids nearly forty miles in length.

Our body takes in an average of five and a half pounds of food and drink each day, which amounts to one ton of solid and liquid nourishment annually. So in seventy years a man or woman eats and drinks 1000 times his or her weight.

There is not known in all the realms of architecture or mechanics one little device which is not found in the human organism. The pulley, the lever, the inclined plane, the hinge, the "universal joint," tubes and trapdoors, the scissors, grindstone, whip, arch, girders, filters, valves, bellows, pump, camera, harp, irrigation plant, telegraph and telephone

146

systems. All these and a hundred other devices which man thinks he has invented, but which have only been telegraphed to the brain from the Solar Plexus and crudely copied or manifested on the objective canvas.

No waterway on earth is so complete or so populous as that wonderful river of life, the blood stream.

It has been said that "all roads lead to Rome." I have discovered that all roads of real knowledge, real health and real fitness lead to the river of life -- the blood. The blood is an epitome of the universe. When man turns the mighty searching's of reason and investigation within the river of life, a new heaven and earth will appear.

While it is true that all body cells are made by the transmutation of blood. It is also true that blood is made from the food and supplements that we eat and the liquids that we drink. The twelve cell or tissue salts with the living anatomical elements—the microzymas—contained in green foods and green drinks are set free by the process of digestion and carried into the circulation through the delicate micro-villi of the small intestine. Air breathed into the lungs enters into the arteries and chemically unites with the cell salts and living anatomical microzymas, and by a wonderful transformation creates blood which then through transmutation creates flesh, bone, muscle, nerves, organs, hair, nails, even a new brain, liver, heart or pancreas.

The quality of the food we eat, the supplements we take, the liquids we drink and the movement or exercising that we engage in determines the quality of the blood. As is the blood, so is the physical, emotional and spiritual body. So is the body, so is the brain. As is the brain, so is the quality of thought. As a man or woman buildeth, so is he or she. And as a man or woman IS, so thinks he or she.

Is there any better way to build blood than with the pH Miracle Lifestyle and Diet that are at the foundation of building the perfect man or the perfect woman? I perceive not.

If you sick or tired with sugar intolerances, if you are weak and overweight from over-acidity, I truly believe there is no better way to build your blood and then your body, mind and spirit, then through these four cornerstone principals of your House of Health:

147

1. Superhydrating with green drinks
2. An alkalizing and energizing diet that includes liberal amounts of green food and healthy fats,
3. An alkalizing and energizing nutritional supplement program, and
4. An alkalizing and energizing exercise and fitness program for body, mind and spirit.

The Wrong Type of Exercise Can Be Hazardous to Your Health!

There is this idea in the fitness and body building world that in order to build strength, size and/or endurance you need to go to the threshold of pain. It has been said, "No pain, No gain!" This, my friend is a philosophy or recipe for disaster, especially when dealing with cancer. To understand why, we need to understand the significance of:

1. The significance of understanding the acid/alkaline balance when exercising
2. The significance of cellular respiration or fermentation during aerobic and anaerobic exercise
3. The significance of fat burning vs. sugar burning and how to tell the difference
4. The significant role of the lymphatic system and skin during exercise
5. The types of exercising and body building activities that are alkalizing and energizing for the body, mind and spirit, especially for the cancer patient, and
6. Additional nutritional supplementation that will support the acid/alkaline balance when exercising.

The Significance of Understanding Acid/Alkaline Balance When Exercising

Anatomically and physiologically the body is an incredible machine that is designed and meant to move. In order to make a signal movement the body needs energy and that energy is created by trillions of anatomical

148

elements, microzymas, that make up the energy factories of every cell, called mitrochondria. It is theorized that within these mitrochondria needed energy is produced for caring out every body function. When a combustion engine burns or ferments fuel to create energy for a car a toxin or acid is released called carbon monoxide. When the mitrochondria of the cell burns or ferments fuel a toxin or acid is released called carbon dioxide. The type of toxin or acid that is release is determined by two important factors:

1. The type of fuel being burned, and
2. The environment in which that fuel is being burned.

For example: when a sprinter is running a 100 meter race he or she is burning sugar for energy producing a less toxic acid carbon dioxide which is expelled through the lungs. When the sprinter takes in less oxygen that is needed he or she becomes oxygen deficient and the mode of energy production changes from respiration (meaning in the presence of oxygen) to fermentation (in the absence of oxygen) producing a more toxic acid, lactic acid that is expelled into the tissues. In order for the body's internal fluids to maintain that delicate pH balance of 7.365 it takes 20 parts of oxygen or bicarbonate to neutralize 1 part carbonic acid or carbon dioxide. That is why you would surely pass out or even die if you stopped breathing for just a few minutes. After the sprinter finishes the race he or she is usually bend over holding his or her knees or lying down gasping for needed oxygen to neutralize the excess build up of acid from the race and regain alkaline balance before passing out or dying. The body will do whatever it has to do to maintain the delicate pH balance of the blood at 7.365 at the cost of expelling acids, like lactic acid, into the tissues. This is when we feel pain. And anytime you experience or feel aches, pain or suffer from irritation or inflammation you are feeling the affect of acid. Therefore acid equals pain and pain equals acid. When you exercise to exhaustion you are creating excess acids that lead to all sickness and disease, including cancer. Acids burn and break down cells that causes a rise in blood sugar. This rise in blood sugar can be devastating to the cancer patient and why exercising to exhaustion or what is called anaerobic exercise or exercising without oxygen can be hazardous to ones health. The fitness and body building ideology of "No Pain, No GAIN" is a scientific illusion. The saying should really say, "With Pain (Acid), No (Healthy) Gain."

It is important to realize that the most important reason for exercising is to eliminate acids from the body via the lungs through respiration or the skin through perspiration. That is why we have two lungs, not one and 3,500 perspiratory pores on our skin per square inch. Exercise moves acids through these two elimination organs reducing endogenous acidity in order to maintain the integrity of all your cells. So when your internal context or environment is alkaline your cells are stronger and healthier and when they are stronger and healthier than your muscles are stronger and healthier, your heart is stronger and healthier, your pancreas is stronger and healthier, every organ and every organ system can function at its optimum level in a balanced pH environment without pain. In fact, in a perfect alkaline state your microzymas, which can never die, would remain in their current healthy cellular state and never break down or theoretically die. What I am suggesting, is life and death is a choice and the choices you make determines the outcomes of your physical and emotional life. Cancer cells live indefinitely in a cup of coffee at 5.5 pH. Cancer cells breakdown in an alkaline pH of 8.0 or above. A healthy human cell could live indefinitely in an alkaline state of 7.365 pH.

When you over exercise or exercise anaerobically you put 75 trillion cells in your body at risk, not for gain, but for loss. Look at some of the athletes we assumed to be healthy and fit, like Jim Fix, the marathon runner or the sprinter Florence Joyner-"Flo Jo," who prematurely died from a heart attack. You hear about athletes every year who die suddenly on or off the track, field or court. The May 19th, 2003, Newsweek cover story on "Treating Pain" states that pain is the number 1 reason Americans visit the doctor at an economic cost of $100 billion a year. Over 10 million children suffer in America from chronic and acute pain that is leading to the increase in childhood diabetes. Why? It is incredibly simple. The cause is over-acidity in the blood and tissues, due to an inverted way of living, eating and thinking, leads to pain, suffering and even death. It is the cause of heart disease. It is the cause of cancer. It is the cause of diabetes. It is the cause of sudden unexplainable death. It is the cause of all sickness and disease. It is the cause of obesity and it is the cause of muscular breakdown or atrophy. It is the cause of all pain and suffering!

On the other hand you have an athlete like Ultra Marathon runner and world record holder Stu Mittleman who ran across American in 57 days doing the equivalent of 2 marathons a day, every day for 57 days without the side affects of excess acid. He understood the importance of burning fat rather than sugar and drank his greens and drank his purred green soups with avocadoes and other good fats while he ran healthfully across America. The idea of carbohydrate loading before a physical event is physiological suicide. In his book, "Slow Burn," Stu Mittleman teaches the significance and importance of burning fat rather than sugar in life and in exercising.

In Chapter (?)-you learned that burning fat produces twice the energy with half the acid production vs. sugar or protein metabolism that creates twice the acid with half the energy production. This is significant when you are trying increase energy and move acids out of the body at the same time. The key to healthful exercise, especially for the cancer patient is Never Go To Pain. If you're in pain you're burning sugar and you're in a state of acidosis or "The Cycle of Imbalance." Stop exercising immediately. Begin immediately hydrating with a green drink and pH drops! Here are a few of the physical and emotional signs of burning sugar vs. fat:

1. You are light headed
2. You are dizzy
3. Your thinking becomes cloudy
4. Your hands or feet are cold
5. You have tingling in your extremities
6. Your peripheral vision narrows
7. You can hear yourself breathing
8. You are inhaling and exhaling through your mouth instead of your nose
9. When running or jogging you become disconnected with your environment. You cannot hear the sound of your feet hitting the road
10. You have a burning sensations in your body
11. You cannot carry on a conversation while exercising
12. Your brow is furrowed and tight
13. Your fists are tight
14. Your muscles are tight

15. You have a knot in your throat
16. You become agitated or are anxiety ridden
17. Your sweat smells like ammonia
18. You are experiencing systemic or localized pain in your body, just to name a few.

In comparison when you are burning fat vs. sugar you will experience the following physical and emotional signs:

1. You have a peaceful feeling
2. You feel grounded
3. You feel connected to your external environment
4. You feel no pain
5. You have a sense of euphoria
6. Your mind is clear
7. You can carry on a conversation while your are exercising
8. Your facial expressions are relaxed and happy
9. Your peripheral vision is widened
10. All your senses are enhanced: vision, hearing, sound, etc.
11. You are inhaling and exhaling through your nose not your mouth
12. Your breathing is quite and easy
13. You will feel more flexible
14. You feel in the zone

Choosing to burn fat as your main source of fuel for energy in life and especially during exercise will minimize acidity, increase energy and vitality, increase strength and endurance, improve the performance of all bodily functions and will extend the quality and quantity of your life. In 2001, I conducted a 6 month study at the United States Army Academy at West Point with the gymnastic team using an alkalizing green drink and pH drops. During the 6 months, all the participants noticed an increase in energy, a decrease in acidity or lactic acid build up after work outs and meets, a decrease in the recovery time after workouts and meets and a notable increase in their performance.

Exercising aerobically without pain will help you remove endogenous acids from your body fluids and tissues and will help provide the

152

alkaline context or terrain for the regeneration and healthy function of all body systems, especially the exocrine and endocrine system. You can now begin the process, Back to the House of Health.

The Significant Role of the Lymphatic System and Skin

Have you ever wonder why you lose tone and strength or experience muscle atrophy when you stop exercising? When you stop exercising your lymphatic system cannot move or vacuum the built up acidity in the tissues so the acids begin tenderizing your muscles like Heinz 57 sauce tenderizes a steak. Acids will turn a body's muscles and organs to mush if one does not move their body. And the best way to move the body is with regular aerobic exercise. When you move your muscles you pump the lymphatic system which in turn pulls or vacuum's the acids, like lactic acid, out of the tissues.

Most people if you ask, have no idea what that lymphatic system is, let alone what it does. So what is the Lymphatic System? The Lymphatic System is a Secondary Circulatory System that follows the blood. Wherever, blood vessels go, so goes the lymphatic vessels. The blood goes out to the cells and back, however the lymph fluid only moves one way, towards the heart. Unlike the Circulatory System, the Lymphatic system lacks a pump to propel the lymph. It relies on new lymph pushing the old lymph and pressure changes in the thoracic duct caused by respiration (breathing, especially deep breathing). Muscular activity, like regular exercise generates a massaging action that stimulates the flow of lymph in the lymphatic vessels. Here are a few important facts to understand:

- Everything you eat or drink goes into the digestive system and ends up in the small intestines
- The intestinal villi have lymphatic lacteals. They both absorb all your nutrition and take it out into the blood stream and lymph to feed and bring nutrients to your cells
- Like an ocean tide, the liquids bath all of your cells and tissues
- Blood and Lymphatic capillaries receive back the fluids to further filter, and detox them from acidic toxins and cellular debris and send them to the lungs, liver, kidneys and skin for excretion.

The lymphatic system is an accessory route to:

1. Remove excess fluid, acids and debris away from the cells. The debris consists of blood proteins, fat globules, pigment, granules, bacteria, yeast, mold, fragmented cells, other debris and waste from chemical reactions within the cells.

2. The lymphatic system is responsible for breaking down the debris in the lymph nodes. In essence the Lymphatic system is responsible for keeping your cells and the surrounding context free of acids and debris which would prevent cells from receiving essential oxygen and nutrients. Removing the excess fluid helps to eliminate swelling and fluid retention. About 80-98% of what leaks out of the blood stream is recovered by the blood capillaries. That leaves 2-20% to find another method of rejoining the blood stream. The lymphatic system is the answer.

3. The Lymphatic System is responsible for returning to the blood, proteins and other substances that have escaped from the blood. The liquid components of blood do not stay within the blood vessels but tend to leak out through the spaces between the cells that make up the walls of capillaries, the smallest blood vessels. Lymph is the fluid which filters out of the bloodstream and when present in excess amounts is know as edema. This fluid accumulates at a rapid rate and if there were no mechanism for its return to the bloodstream, we would die in about twenty-four hours from circulatory failure.

4. The fluid volume and pressure in the tissues is regulated by the lymphatic system.

5. The Lymphatic System transfers digested fat from the intestine to the bloodstream.

6. The lymph helps to transport lymphocytes and other immuno-competent cells throughout the body.

7. The lymph nodes produce lymphocytes.

Part of the Body's Janitorial Service Science refers to as the Immune System

The Janitorial System or Immune System and the Lymphatic System work in concert together to keep the body free from acidic toxins, biological transmutations, like bacteria and yeast, and other cellular debris like cell fragments. Lymph fluid houses white blood cells which produce antibodies to bind to antigens or microforms and acids.

The Structure/Function of the Lymphatic System

The Lymphatic System is very similar to the run-off of a mountain after a rain storm. As the water starts to run down hill it follows no pattern. The small trickles are very random and are never the same. The trickles (lymphatic capillaries) join together into little streams (lymphatic vessels) and they become larger and larger until they are rivers and often enter ponds and lakes (lymph nodes). The rivers join the ocean (the bloodstream) for the process to start again.

Lymph is the clear fluid that bathes the cells of the body. In these interstitial spaces the lymph is constantly interacting with the blood capillaries. The lymph surrounding the cells helps the blood to deliver nutrients, eliminate acid waste and enables the exchange of oxygen and carbon dioxide. Lymph is plasma that has moved from the blood into the interstitial spaces or the spaces around the cells. It contains very few red blood cells, less protein and oxygen than blood plasma and has a high content of white blood cells, especially lymphocytes. It is very similar in substance to sinovial fluid which lubricates the joints. Lymph fluid is also called interstitial fluid or tissue fluid. It is classified as a tissue fluid because of the number of living cells it contains.

Lymphatic capillaries are the beginning of the lymphatic system. They begin blindly in the interstitial spaces where the lymph fluid drains into them. Lymphatic capillaries allow larger molecules, like blood proteins, to pass through their walls. The only place that lymphatic capillaries are not present is in the central nervous system and the brain.

Lymphatic vessels are formed by lymphatic capillaries joining together. They are drainage channels into lymph nodes, catch basins for toxic acids or cellular debris. The body has twice as many lymphatic vessels as blood vessels but their size is much smaller than the blood vessels. Lymph vessels have thinner walls than the veins and have more valves. The one way valves cause a beaded appearance in the vessel. The vessels are lined with a thin, smooth wall of muscle. The lymph is moved forward when the muscles contract when breathing, moving or exercising. The lymphatic vessels lead into the lymph nodes for the lymph fluid to be filtered.

One of the most challenging problems for the physiologist is to explain why lymph vessel walls seem to be permeable in one direction only. Experimentally, bacteria, red blood cells, and graphite particles have been shown to penetrate the lymphatic system without difficulty. Yet once these substances have penetrated, they seem to be retained and to find their way back into the bloodstream via larger ducts without leakage.

Afferent vessels are the vessels leading into the lymph node. There can be many vessels coming in at different locations on the lymph node. Efferent vessels are the vessels that leave the lymph node after filtration of the lymph fluid.

The lymph nodes vary in size and shape from a hemp-seed to an almond shape. The body can have between 400 and 1,000 lymph nodes. Half are in the abdomen region and around the organs of the body. These catch basins for cellular debris and acids embody a large numbers of leukocytes embedded in a network of connective tissue. The lymph fluid being returned to the bloodstream passes through several lymph nodes. The lymph nodes are check stations for the lymphatic system. They filter and purify the lymph from cellular debris and acids. They act as a quarantine for noxious acidic products of inflammatory or malignant lesions and then breakdown those products. They reabsorb some of the water, because the lymph is 95% water, thus concentrating it. They produce lymphocytes which are released into the blood for janitorial support. When the production level of lymphocytes in the lymph nodes is increased and released into the blood to clean-up acid waste and cellular debris, the lymph node begins to swell.

The lymph nodes serve as a center for the production of phagocytes (white blood cells that collect garbage), which engulf bacteria and acidic poisonous substances. During the course of any excess acidity from lifestyle or diet, the lymph nodes become enlarge because of the large number of phagocytes being produced; these lymph nodes are often painful and inflamed because of the acidity and cellular debris. The swollen glands most often observed are located on the neck, in the armpit, and in the groin.

Lymph nodes are divided into several compartments which contain white cells or lymphocytes. If the lymph node cannot cope with the increased acidity and/or cellular debris, outfection will set into the lymph nodes and the acidic fluid will enter the blood compromising the delicate pH balance of the blood.

Bottom line, the lymphatic system is the vacuum cleaner of the tissues and blood and is responsible for keeping the internal fluids of the body free from excess acidity, biological transmutations and other cellular debris. When you over-exercise and build up lactic acid in the tissue it is the lymphatic system that cleans the acidity out of the tissue. This is why you see runners or even race horses take an extra lap before stopping, helping to move lactic acid build-up out of the tissue. Always remember if you are feeling any pain in the body then you are feeling localized acidity that can only be removed by and through the lymphatic system.

What are the causes lymphatic system blockage?

1. Large-molecule proteins produced as a result of tissue breakdown

2. Acidic foods like beef, chicken, pork, eggs, protein drinks, high sugar foods, processed fats and foods not properly digested

3. Lack of regular aerobic exercise-lymphatic fluid relies on movement of the muscles to remove cellular debris and excess acid

4. Toxic chemicals-medications, preservatives etc.

5. Anger-when we become angry our bodies produce acids that are toxic to our bodies, capillaries dilate and release blood proteins which are too big to enter back into the blood stream

6. Cellular waste from chemical reactions in the cells

7. Other by-products that cannot be picked up by blood stream, such as trapped blood proteins, and,

8. Acid build up when the lymphatic system slows down due to stress, fatigue, lack of physical activity, over exercise or anaerobic excercise, certain food additives and emotional shock.

What happens when the lymphatic system is sluggish or blocked?

1. Pain from acidic buildup due to lack of oxygen to the cells
2. Lower levels of efficiency in the body
3. Blocked circulation due to acid build up
4. Fluid retention to neutralize acidic build up
5. Cellular displacement
6. Systemic and localized pain from acid build up
7. Loss of energy from acid build up
8. Degenerative disease, like cancer, and even death due to excess acidity

All pain as mentioned earlier is caused by unoxygenated cells and tissues that leads to cellular breakdown and the expression of debilitating acids. Pain always is an indication of acid build up in the tissues and blockages in the lymphatic system.

When the lymph slows down the cell is suspended in an acidic moat. Fresh oxygen and fuel (glucose or fats) cannot get to the cell. The glucose then ferments creating toxic acids in the interstitial spaces causing the body cells to begin their biologically transmutation because of the lack of oxygen and a compromised pH environment. The biological transformed cells have a ferocious appetite for sugar and feed on the fermented glucose. This is the beginning stages of sugar intolerance that leads to cancer. If and when the lymphatic system cleans out the acid moat then and only then can oxygen and glucose get into the cell for cellular energy. This is a critical point for the cancer patient to understand and why regular healthful aerobic exercise is so important. When you move your body through regular aerobic exercise, you pump lymphatic vessels that vacuum's and pulls out acidic toxins and cellular debris in the tissues left behind by the blood from sugar and protein metabolism, which in turn leads to a more alkaline environment in the tissues and a healthier and energized body.

The types of exercising and body building activities that are alkalizing and energizing for the body, mind and spirit, especially when dealing with cancer

There are several passive forms of exercise that are excellent for moving the lymphatic fluids that in turn will reduce endogenous acidity, leading to outstanding health and fitness. The first is a specialized kind of massage called the Lymphatic massage.

Claire Maxwell Hudson describes the Benefits of Massage in her book "The complete book of massage." She states, "a massage has profound effects on the health of the person being massaged. It improves circulation, relaxes muscles, aids digestion and, by stimulating the lymphatic system, speeds up the elimination of waste products. These direct benefits of feeling cared for and cosseted, quickly produce a marvelous feeling of well-being that cannot be matched by modern drugs."

The lymphatic system was recognized as early as the Greeks who named the lymph in the lacteals (which are lymphatic capillaries in the intestines). Hippocrates correlated ill health to lymphatic temperament.

Dr. Emil Vodder a European Physical Therapist developed Manual Lymph Drainage. An excerpt, from Dr. William N. Brown, Ph.D., N.D., D. Sc., from "The Touch that Heals, The secret key to strengthening the immune system," he states, "wouldn't it be wonderful if we could just walk into our doctor's office and say, I want you to increase my body's ability to use nutrients, balance my hormones, reduce my level of stress, cleanse my body, strengthen my immune system, and do it all in one hour! Sound far fetched? Not at all, because all of this can be accomplished with lymphatic manipulation. This revolutionary technique is an immune strengthening gentle massage, developed in Europe in the 1930's by Dr. Emil Vodder of Denmark. Refinement of Lymphatic Manipulation by Dr. Asdonk, in a clinic in the Black Forest region of Germany, and research done by Foldi, Mislin, and others have proven the effectiveness of this technique. This modality is fully accepted by the medical insurance plans in Europe and doctors write prescriptions for this treatment on a routine basis there. (This technique

159

was refined and improved by Dr. Vodder's Student, Dr. Anita Childs). I studied lymphatic Manipulation with Dr. Childs, and have practiced it for over 12 years with excellent results. These results are even greater when combined with holistic nutritional therapy."

The Benefits of Lymphatic Massage

Lymphatic massage will move acidity from sugar and protein metabolism and thus help or even eliminate the following symptomologies:

Edema
Toxicity
Swelling
Fibromyalgia
Tenderness or over sensitivity to touch
Leg Cramps
Carpal Tunnel Syndrome
Tennis elbow
Sciatica
Stress
Tired and overworked muscles.
Bursitis
Multiple Sclerosis
Cellulite (in combination with health eating habits and exercise)
Headaches
Anxiety
Recovery from injuries and surgery with less scarring

When muscles are overworked they produce lactic acid. After a lymphatic massage the acids and waste material surrounding the muscle is removed and the muscle has more power because of increased efficiency. This also means that the acids in or around the tissues of the body are also eliminated. Lymphatic massage can increase recovery and/or healing time by 30% and there is 30% less scarring.

After the massage it is normal to feel sluggish, foggy, fatigued and nauseated. This is due to the amount of acids that were in the stagnant fluid in the tissues that are now be handled by your body. Drinking your green drink or alkalized and energized water will help your body to rid itself of the acidic toxins.

160

Why Lymphatic Massage is different

Lymphatic Massage is different from other modalities of massage because:

1. The massage therapist pumps the lymph nodes
2. The massage therapist works toward the lymph nodes, and
3. The massage therapist works in the connective tissue that houses the lymphatic vessels

The main lymph nodes the massage therapist pumps are at the clavicle, the axillary, in the armpit, the cubital, the bend of the arm, inguinal, the bend of the hip and popliteal, the backside of the knee. The pumping of the lymph nodes is similar to the primer on a lawn mower. When the primer bulb is compressed the gas in the primer is pushed toward the engine. When the primer is released, the bulb expands and creates suction to pull the gas from the tank into the bulb. Applying pressure to the lymph node pushes the lymph in the node toward the heart. When the pressure is released, the node expands, pulling the lymph into the node. This increases the lymph flow in the body.

The lymphatic vessels have one way valves that go toward lymph nodes. If you apply pressure away from the heart you cause a back flow in the lymphatic system. I have heard it said that working away from the heart increases blood flow. However, the arteries are very deep and close to the bone making it difficult to work on them. The arteries carrying the blood have incredible power because the blood has just been pumped from the heart and working with the effects of gravity. The veins returning to the heart are closer to the surface making them very accessible. They also have one way valves and are going against gravity. These veins need the assistance of massage.

Lymphatic massage is achieved by massaging the lymphatic vessels in the connective tissues that holds muscle to the bone. Because the Lymphatic system has no pump to move the fluid it relies on motion produced by muscles being active, breathing, and arteries. Lymphatic massage is an outside force that moves the stagnated lymph through the vessels and allows the fresh lymph to occupy the space.

What you can do to help your Lymphatic System help maintain the delicate pH balance of the body fluids at 7.365

1. Deep Breathing is very important to release and eliminate acidic toxins and increase lymphatic flow. When the lymph and its acidic toxins are deposited into the bloodstream the first organ they reach are the lungs. Deep breathing will help to expel these acidic toxins so your lymphatic system doesn't have to work as hard.

2. Participate in passive or low impact aerobic exercise that stimulates the Lymphatic and Circulatory System like:

   a. Walking is a great way to get the muscles moving to pump the lymphatic fluids moving acids out of the tissue and increasing circulation. I always suggest walking long enough or far enough until you break a sweat. Sweating is one of the best reasons for exercising and is an excellent way to move acidic gases and fluids out of the body through the third kidney, the skin. It usually takes approximately 20 minutes for a man to begin sweating and 30 minutes for a woman. When walking stay relaxed and aware of everything around you and make sure you are breathing in and out through your nose.

   b. Jogging should be done with prudence and understanding. One of the biggest mistakes that joggers or runners make, according to world record holder and long distance runner, Stu Mittleman, is in the size of the shoes worn. For example, my dress shoe size is 9 to 9 ½ but my jogging shoe size is 10 ½. The reason for the larger shoe is to give your feet the room they need as the foot rolls forward the foot spreads requiring more room. If the needed room is not there because the shoe size is too small this will cause irritation, inflammation, sores, pain, blood blisters, in-grown toe nails, etc., from always banging the toes into the front part of the shoe. More good information on how to jog or run aerobically can be in Stu Mittleman's book, "Slow Burn" published by Harper Collins.

162

Jogging should be a pleasurable experience not a painful one and should always be aerobic not anaerobic. If you begin experiencing any pain while jogging slow down and walk for awhile until the pain subsides. Always remember to breathe in and out through your nose not your mouth. And the most important part of the jog is to sweat which means you have increased blood and lymphatic circulation and thus reduced systemic acidosis. And when you reduce acidity you improve health and fitness through maintaining the delicate pH balance of the internal body fluids.

c. Swimming is one of the best low impact aerobic forms of exercise. The only draw back to swimming every day is the availability of a lap pool.

d. Yoga is the oldest of the physical disciples. According to the Pilates Method Plus by Jennifer Kries, "It is an immortal art, science and philosophy. It is the true union of ones will with spirituality-the disciplining of the intellect, the emotions, the body and the mind. Yoga also offers a balancing element emphasis not found in Pilates but Pilates and Yoga alike they both focus on the mind, body as a integrated whole." Yoga is good for many symptomologies, including cancer. Yoga improves muscle tone, flexibility, strength and stamina, reduces tension and improves circulation and oxygenation through breath, boosts self-esteem, improves concentration through mind body awareness, lowers fat, stimulates the janitorial service and gives you a sense of overall well-being through calming the nervous system.

e. Pilates

f. Resistance weight training is technically referred to as "high-intensity, low-force exercise" according to former top professional bodybuilder Mike Mentzer,, in his book, "Muscles in Minutes." He suggests, "Using weights that allow for the performance of 6 to 15 repetitions is low-to-moderate force. As long as you perform the suggested exercises in a controlled, slow manner, the forces will never exceed those imposed by the actual resistance. This form of exercise is perfectly safe-far safer than jogging or almost any other exercise activity." To gain maximum benefit from resistance weight training you need to understand the word failure. By way of illustration, let's assume you are doing barbell curls with 30 pounds, and you just completed the eighth repetition with considerable effort. Continue to try to perform the ninth, and if you can't lift the weight completely to the top, cease immediately. You have completed the exercise. You have also created through the resistance a positive energy field, around the bicep muscle that attracts the flow of blood to the bicep, due to the blood's negative electrical surface charge. As the blood flows into the positive energy field, this is where and when the blood biologically transmutates into new muscle cells to support the new stress created by the resistance training. This is why you can create new muscles not only in minutes but in seconds. Keep in mind, that this is the theory of the "New Biology." This theory suggests that it is the blood that becomes muscle and the quality of the muscle is determined by the quality of the blood and the quality of the blood is determined by the quality and quantity of green foods and green drinks in your diet. The size and strength of any muscle is not determined by the quality or quantity of protein one is eating but by the quality and quantity of high chlorophyll foods one is eating to build strong blood cells. All of the strongest animals in the world are a witness to this theory of a diet high in chlorophyll content foods.

Another good book on resistance weight training is "Static Contraction" by Peter Sisco and John Little. The authors suggest lifting a weight and holding that weight statically for a period of only 15 seconds at two or three inches below lockout (strongest range), and held there without any up or down motion. Intensity is increased by progressively holding the weight for longer periods of time. After 15 seconds the weight would begin to descend or ascend, in the case of a lat pulldown or similar movement. When a weight could be held for 30 seconds, the weight is then increased sufficiently so that the person could hold the weight for only 15 seconds, and the progression would start over again. Static Contraction weight training creates a positive energy field at the point just below lockout which then attracts the flow of blood to this point of stress causing a biological transmutation of blood cells to muscle cells to support the increased weight. This is how you create muscles in seconds without overstressing the body. The greater the intensity applied during training, the greater the growth stimulation and the briefer the workout. I refer to this type of weight training more accurately as static attraction because of the opposite energy fields or poles created in the body during the training. I perceive the objective in building muscles should never be to see how much exercise you can tolerate, but rather just how little exercise is required to stimulate and create a static attraction whereby increase in muscle size and strength can be accomplished.

This same phenomenon happens when the body is injured, such as in a broken bone or a cut. When measuring the energy fields at the break or the cut you will find a positive energy field of approximately, positive 8 to 10 millivolts. As blood flow increases to the break or cut as a result of static attraction, the energy field changes to a negative 8 to 10 millivolts. It is in this energy field of negative 8 to 10 millivolts that the blood biologically transmutates to skin, bones, nerve cells, etc., that brings about the healing or regeneration of the bone or the healing of the cut. When the regeneration or healing has taken place the bioenergy fields revert back to their normal energy field of negative 1, millivolts.

The beauty of resistance weight training is you only need to be in the gym for 20 to 30 minutes at the most. After the break-in period which lasts for about two weeks the amount of time in the gym will reduce to about 10 to 15 minutes. The principal of "less is more and more is less and less more often is better than more less often" applies

165

here to resistant training. Further, you do not need to take supplemental protein in your diet to build muscles. Muscle cells are built from blood not protein and blood is built with green foods and green drinks. But, before starting any weight training program please consult with your physician first.

g. Acupuncture or Acupressure creates a point of stress know as piezoelectricity or a positive energy field. This positive energy field created by the needle or the finger or hand pressure causes an increase of blood flow and a static attraction to the positive pole or the point of the needle or pressure. For the same reasons as mentioned above the blood will biologically transmutate into new body cells to facilitate healing and regeneration in the area of the body that is stressed. This is why acupuncture and acupressure can be helpful for anyone who is sick and tired, or challenged with a chronic condition like cancer.

h. Jumping on mini Trampoline like the Cellerciser. According to David Hall the creator of Cellercise, he states, "Cellercising uses a vertical movement like weight lifting, push-ups, pull-ups or sit-ups in a repetitive up-and-down motion. However, these conventional forms of exercise target and isolate specific muscles or muscle groups making it very time consuming, often tearing down and damaging the body to build it up. Cellercising flexes all 75 trillion cells at the same time!" Even better, it requires on 15 minutes twice a day.

Unlike jogging, walking, bicycling, weightlifting, cellercising is isotonic, isometric, calisthenic and aerobic all in one:

1. Isotonic: moving up and down on the cellerciser is full body weight bearing activity and strengthens muscles, connective tissue, ligaments and bones.

2. Isometric: by altering the angle of the body, specific cells resist "G-Forces." This tightens, lifts and tones internal organs, muscles, even skin cells.

166

3. Calisthenic: is another form of resistance training that uses your own body weight to create the static attraction rather than free weights or machines. There are different techniques that can be used to target every part of the body, including thighs, knees, hips, buttocks, waist, stomach, arms, chin, and intestines.

4. Aerobic: for 15 minutes, twice a day, you can challenge every cell in you cardiovascular pulmonary system.

Cells expand and contract through vertical, or up-and-down movement on the Cellerciser. This movement creates a cellular massage to increase circulation, improve lymphatic drainage, break up lymphatic blockages, open blood vessels, and strengthen the cell membrane. Healthy and strong cells are more resistant to cellular breakdown. During Cellercise, all 75 trillion cells flex nearly 100 times per minute, cell by cell, strengthening the body from the inside out.

According to Dr. Morton Walker, in his article, "Don't Exercise, Cellercise" he states the following, "Cellercise provides a stimulus for free-flowing lymphatics which drain away potential poisons from the cells. Unlike the arterial blood supply system, the lymphatic vessels do not own their own pump. They have no heart muscle to move the lymph fluid through their transfer channels. Muscular contraction, gravitational pressure, and internal massage of the lymph duct valves activate the flow of lymph away from tissue and back to the main pulmonary circulation. Cellercising supplies all three methods and blood enters the capillaries, supplying the cells with fresh fluid containing food and oxygen. The bouncing motion moves and recycles lymph and blood through the circulatory system many times during the course of a cellercising session and promotes a healthier bodily environment."

One of the more valuable exercises performed in the cellercising program is a twisting motion. "The effect of this twisting action on the digestive system is significant," says Lawrence R. Stowe, Ph.D., of Atlanta, Georgia. "It is difficult, if not impossible, to exercise the smooth muscles of the intestinal tract. These muscles are needed for elimination of digestive waste. But even these muscles receive a daily tune-up with cellercise."

Here are twenty-five reasons for Cellercising at least twice a day for 10 to 15 minutes:

1. Increased balance and coordination

2. Reduced chances of cardiovascular challenges

3. Increased production of red blood cells

4. Aid in lymphatic circulation

5. Strengthen heart and other muscles in the body

6. Lower resting heart rate

7. Reduces cholesterol and triglyceride levels

8. Increased stimulation of metabolism

9. Improved vision

10. Increased heart capacity

11. Greater circulation and increased oxygenation to the tissue

12. Increased thyroid output

13. Expanded body capacity for fuel storage

14. Increased muscle vigor and tone muscle fiber

15. Reduced aches and pains from lack of exercise

16. Reduced headaches and back pains

17. Improved digestion and elimination

18. Improved sleep and relaxation

19. Improved mental performance

20. Keener learning processes

21. Less fatigue and menstrual discomfort

22. Improved janitorial service or white cell activity

23. Improved glandular function

24. Loss of excess weight.

According to Paul E. DeVore, M.D. advised that cellercising uses calories eleven times faster than walking, five times faster than swimming, and three times faster than running. He also suggested that cellercising burns calories more efficiently than other forms of movement because all the body's cells are using energy simultaneously. Instead of flexing muscles, Cellercising is squeezing and releasing acidic products from every single cell resulting in elimination of excess water and waste.

I believe that daily Cellercising is one of the best low impact aerobic activities for young and old that you can do anytime in the convenience of your own home that eliminates up to 80% of the impact on the bones and joints and at the same time moves acids out of the tissues from sugar and protein metabolism by activating the lymphatic system. This in turn provides for a cleaner internal environment and a healthy and fit body. For the cancer patient, Cellercising is one of the most important daily activities in boosting your immune-fighting cells and your overall immune system. For more information on Cellercising, go to www.thephmiracle.us.

i. The Cross Trainer is another excellent low impact aerobic exercise apparatus that works the lower and upper body in a back and forth forward movement, like walking or jogging. This equipment has several settings that regulates time of exercise, speed of exercise, distance, heart rate, resistance on both legs and arms and the type of terrain the exercise can take place, whether level or up and down. I recommend at least 30 minutes a day starting out on the lowest settings. I have personally found the Life Fitness Cross Trainer to be the best all round cross trainer. You can find the Life Fitness Cross Trainer in most good gyms.

3. Self massage-always rub toward the heart. When massaging you must always move your hands towards the heart to increase the lymphatic flow.

4. Body Brushing- Using a brush on dry skin working toward the heart to help your lymphatics. When body brushing or self-massaging work the area immediately around the lymph node first, then always apply pressure toward the node. Work your way away from the node. Similar to working a snarl in your hair, you would work the end, clear that area then work the next section and up until the snarl is cleared.

5. Dry Heat Sauna is one of the best passive exercises because the of the radiant heat of an infrared sauna causes a profound deep sweat. Because of the level of pollution we are exposed to and its many sources, as well as poor dietary and exercise habits, the therapeutic value of regular sweating has become immense. It has benefits for body, mind and spirit, which are the primary benefits of exercise. After about 30 minutes of exposure, the blood vessels of the skin dilate to allow more blood to flow to the surface to support the cooling process. The millions of glands covering the body are infused with fluid from the blood. IN turn, they empty to the skin's surface, thereby flushing large amounts of toxins, including toxic acids and heavy metals, from the body.

My research over the years has shown that a radiant heat sauna provides the following benefits:

* Speeds up metabolic processes of vial organs and glands, including the endocrine glands, like the pancreas.

* Inhibits the development of pleomorphic microforms and creates a "fever reaction" of rising temperature that removes their acidic wastes.

* Increases the number of leukocytes or white blood cells in the blood to help clean up the internal terrain.

* Places demand on the heart to work harder, thus exercising it and also producing a drop in diastolic blood pressure (the low side).

170

* Stimulates the dilation of peripheral blood vessels, thus relieving pain (including muscle pain) and speeding the healing of sprain, bursitis, arthritis, and peripheral vascular conditions.

* Creates a positive energy field (static attraction) on the surface of the skin causing greater blood circulation and thus the removal of acidic toxins through the pores of the skin.

* Promotes relaxation, thereby creating a feeling of well-being.

For those who are unable to exercise sufficiently for whatever reason, the radiant heat infrared sauna is an excellent way of getting the benefits of exercise without the undue stress on the skeleton, muscles, and associated tissues. Such people, including cancer patients have an even greater need for exercise, and the sauna fills the bill. It is important to remember that sweating depletes the body of beneficial minerals, therefore it is absolutely crucial to replenish your nutrients with green drinks and pH drops.

6. Drink green drinks and alkalized and energized water as discussed in Chapters 7 and 8. The body is 2/3 water and most of that is lymphatic fluid so you should be drinking at least 4 liters of alkalized and energized fluids a day. It is important to drink at least 4 liters of alkalized water a day because the blood is 96% water. Blood is responsible for feeding and nourishing the cells and picking up the waste from the cells. Blood will service the cells regardless of the amount of water you dink, however if you do not drink enough water you force the blood to rob from the body. This shows up in the mucosum layer of the skin. In Europe they believe that chronic dehydration takes 6-7 years to correct with outside help. Alkalized and energized water also helps the kidneys to flush out the acidic toxins. Because the waste that the lymphatic system picks up is deposited in the blood stream and then filtered in the kidneys this is especially important to drink a green drink or alkalized water after a massage.

7.

7. Supplements & Herbs -When you drink your green drinks they help your body to alkalize the acids that the lymphatic massage or exercise will have stirred up. When the toxins settle around the cells they act as a moat, not allowing food and oxygen to get to the cells. When the lymphatic system is clean the nutrients from the green drink flowing in the blood can be utilized by the cells. To help support and lymphatic system, which also includes the spleen and thymus, I would suggest extra Vitamin A plus a combination of other specific vitamins, minerals, herbs and cell salts, a synergistic herbal nutritional formulation.

Vitamin A is essential for the repair and growth of mucus membranes that line the digestive tract, respiratory tract, salivary glands, tear ducts and eyes, as well as all other cell membranes in the body. Vitamin A helps regulate the formation of cartilage and many hormones. It also aids in the detoxification of acids, has co-enzyme functions in the retina, skin, liver, bone, and adrenal glands. It also helps protect the body during stress from injuries, anxiety, surgery and promotes resistance to outside toxins.

Vitamin A is an essential nutrient the body needs to neutralize acidity. By strengthening the cell walls, it helps to protect the mucous membranes against biological transmutations of bacteria and yeast and their associated exotoxins and mycotxins.

Vitamin A helps to protect the epithelial tissues like the skin, the stomach, and the lungs from becoming over-acidic and breaking down.

Vitamin A is essential in the chemical process of cholesterol conversion into female estrogens and male androgens. An insufficient supply of these sex hormones results in cellular breakdown of the sex organs. When animals in this condition were given Vitamin A they returned to normal hormone activity. Healthy aerobic exercise can also include a healthy sex life which can be enhanced with extra Vitamin A and zinc. Sexual intercourse increases both blood and lymphatic flow helping to move acidity out of the tissues and elimination of those toxins through the skin and other elimination organs.

Fish liver oil is an excellent natural source of Vitamin A. To insure complete absorption and to eliminate the oil intolerance problem some people have, I suggest that three different sources of Vitamin A be used:

1. A dry, water dispersable, relatively oil free fish liver oil source of Vitamin A.

2. A dry, water dispersable , oil free plant source of pro-vitamin A known as carotene, and,

3. A variety of pro-vitamin A containing plants and herbs including wheat grass, barley grass, oat grass, dandelion and parsley.

Some other the other ingredients that are helpful in supporting the lymphatic system and the elimination of acids are:

Octacossanol exists in nature as a bio-chemical of many plant oils, including the oil of raw wheat germ. It is known for its effects on physical fitness such as improving endurance, increased boy reaction time, basal metabolism, oxygen intake and oxygen debt. The use of octacossanol from unrefined, unheated wheat germ oils, because of its unique properties, has gained wide acceptance by athletes and those suffering from heart and circulatory disorders as a result of excess acidity that has localized to those areas of the body.

N-N-Dimethyglycine is a water soluble, tertiary amino protein, non-fuel nutrient. It has been found to have some relationship to choline, an important B-complex vitamin. It can be isolated from food sources such as apricot kernels. Dimenthylglycine is known for its greater efficiency and purity in comparison to its analog or counterpart, calcium pangamate. It has no undesirable side effects and its toxic level for man is 100,000 times the therapeutic dose. In research performed by Dr. Charles D. Graber of the University of South Carolina, School of Medicine, using double blind studies, showed that dimethyglycine enhance both antibody production and cellular immunity in humans using less than 100 mg. per day. The research also found dimethylglcine beneficial as a nutritional support for the following conditions: hardening of the arteries, high levels of cholesterol due to excess acidity, elevated blood pressure, elevated blood sugar, degenerative nerve conditions, abnormal cell development, painful joints and muscles due to localized acidity, and inadequate cellular oxygenation.

173

Superoxide Dismutase or SOD is an excellent anti-acid. Scientific research conducted at Duke University Center, points to the fact that acids (free-radicals) may be associated with the build up of inflammation in the body tissue. Their research led them to the discovery of an anti-inflammatory protein enzyme that they called, "orgotein" which was later named "superoxide dismutase." Therefore, SOD may play an important role in preventing cellular transmutation, neutralizing acid and thus slowing down the aging process.

Research indicates that no more than 50,000 IU per day can be utilized by the body except in therapeutic cases, where up to 100,000 are recommended for short periods of time not to exceed three months. I would suggest that the best level is somewhere between 25,000 and 50,000 IU for the cancer patient weighing 70 kilos or 154 pounds. Each capsule should contain at least 10,000 IU of Beta carotene and fish liver oil. Recommended dosage is 1 capsule with a green drink or alkalized and energized water with pH drops 6 times a day.

In the words of Walt Whitman:

"I loaf and invite my soul; I lean and loaf at my ease, observing a spear of summer grass. Clear and sweet is my soul, and clear and sweet is all that is not my soul."

"Welcome every organ and attribute of me, and of any man hearty and clean, not an inch, not a particle of an inch, is vile, and none shall be less familiar than the rest."

"Divine am I, inside and out, and I make holy whatever I touch or am touched from."

"I say no man has ever yet been half devout enough; none has ever yet adored or worshipped half enough; none has begun to think how divine he himself is, and how certain the future is."

Cancer is not a disease but a symptom of imbalance within. May you realize how certain your future is if you choose wisely and realize that the pathway to the House of Health of ultimate outstanding health and fitness lies from within not from without.

USEFUL RESOURCES

For those who do not have a doctor in their area that is willing to do the IV's, we have a licensed hospital with a staff of licensed medical doctors in Rosarita Baja California. A 50-room hospital right there on the ocean where you can not only enjoy the beautiful scenery which is alkalizing in itself, but also receive the pH Miracle alkalizing program in just an incredible way and have the supervision of doctors and nurses that have been trained in the new biology and in this alkalizing approach-the pH Miracle program-with every meal prepared properly, to the lymphatic massage, to the infrared saunas, to the IV's, to whatever needs to be done in order to move that balance of alkalinity back into your system. Even to providing more oxygen to the overall body through a hyperbaric chamber, oxygen chamber where you actually are infused into an oxygen state to begin the process of re-alkalizing the body. And, as was said by Dr. Warburg, the difference between a cancerous cell and a normal cell is its change of metabolism going from respiration to fermentation. And of course what that means is a cell changes its metabolism from respiration to fermentation when it's in an oxygen deprived state. So the hyperbaric chamber helps to return that oxygen state so the metabolism can take place in a proper way rather than producing *lactic acid* which I believe is one of the major contributors to cancerous tissue.

One of the major food groups that contributes to lactic acid is the sugar lactose which is found in all dairy products. And of course the highest incidences of breast cancer and prostate cancer are found in those areas, those cultures, that eat liberal amounts of dairy products which should never be eaten and should definitely be eliminated out of the diet. Of course any foods or supplements that have lactose in them, and yes you need to get in the habit of reading the labels because there are many supplements that have hidden sugars, these supplements are sweetened up with fructose or anything that has OSE- lactose, fructose, sucrose, anything with OSE in it-you know that that is trouble. You want to move away from all the types of sugar.

You know step seven of the pH Miracle living program is the

175

understanding that all healing starts from the inside out. From the head down and in a reverse order as symptoms have appeared. Let me restate that for you. It can be put like this: All healing starts from the bowel, and we have to go upstream. Of course it starts in the mouth with our base diet, but it starts with the bowels outward. From the brain center to the organs they control in a reverse order as symptoms are stored in memory. You cannot have a healthy body if you do not have healthy bowels. You have to clean up that environment. That pristine area has to be alkalized with the proper foods and liquids that will do that. And this is why this program has to be monitored by those who are trained in the New Biology who understand the process of alkalizing. This is not something you should do on your own, especially if you're dealing with a serious condition. You're not going to get the results. You just don't understand. You're going to have to learn how to do this. That's why we have different points of entry. Yes, you can learn about the program through our books but the pH Miracle retreat is such an easy way to really get indoctrinated and get the understanding because as the scripture says, *knowledge is power*. And as Moses said, *my people perish for lack of knowledge*. We are killing ourselves with what we're eating and what we're drinking and what we're thinking. And if we can make the changes to a more alkalized, energized lifestyle, then we're going to get a different result-rather than sickness and disease, we're going to get health, energy and vitality.

So I invite you to refer to the following list of resources and to go to our website to look at our offering here at our ranch (Rancho Del Sol) and at Sanoviv. And also take a look at all of our literature too as well. If you need pH hydrion paper, for testing the saliva and urine, we have that available on our website. If you need more information, go to articles. It's my goal to provide as much information, free information, and to disseminate that to as many people as we can around the world so they can know the truth of what it takes, what it is, what it feels like, and how easy it can be to have an incredible and extraordinary health, energy and vitality.

RESOURCES

The pH Miracle
pHorever Young
Innerlight, Inc.
The pH Miracle Living Centers
16390 Dia Del Sol
Valley Center, CA 92082
Phone: 760.751.8321, 760.484.8676
Fax: 760.751.8324
www.phmiraclelife@gmail.com, www.phoreveryoung.com,
www.ijuicenow.com, www.innerlightblue.com, www.phwisdom.com
(UK), www.alkalinecare.com (Spain), www.phmiracleretreat.com
(Italy), www.phmlife.com, www.phmiraclestore.com,
www.universalmedicalimaging.com (Los Angeles, California)

Call for referrals for live blood analysis and the Mycotoxic/Oxidative
Stress Test (MOST), or health retreats and consultations, and
information not covered in this section about products mentioned in
this book. Ore check out these websites:
www.drrobertyoung.com or www.phmiracleretreat.com

For general information about Needak rebounders, pH paper, and
more, including workshops on preparing alkalizing meals through
Shelley Young's Academy or Culinary Arts.
www.drrobertyoung.com or www.phmiracleretreat.com

For general information, articles, and testimonials, as well as more
information on the Plasma Activated Electro-Magnetic MicroIonization
Water Machine.
www.phoreveryoung.com and www.ijuicenow.com,
www.innerlightblue.com

For pH Miracle Living Nutritionals (supplements), the Regenesis
Water Machine, videos on the New Biology and the pH Miracle
lifestyle and diet, and information about The pH Miracle Living
Foundation, which is dedicated to children with serious health
challenges, and helping them and their parents with alternative health
education.

www.phoreveryoung.com and www.drrobertyoung.com and www.phmiracleretreat.com

For organically grown California avocados, picked fresh off the tree and shipped to you next day: 760.751.8321; www.phoreveryoung.com and www.phmiracle.com

Extra-virgin coconut oil: Garden of Life, 800-622-8986; www.gardenoflifeusa.com

Heat Wave Seasoning from the Cape Herb and Spice Company, distributed by Profile Products: P.O. Box 140, Maple Valley, WA 98038; 425-432-4300; www.elements-of-spice.com

Spice Hunter Spices
San Luis Obispo, CA 93401
800-444-3061
www.spicehunter.com

Real Salt
Redmond Minerals, Inc.
800-367-7258
www.realsalt.com

InnerLight Biological Research Center
134 E. 200 No.
Alpine, UT 84004
801-756-7850
www.innerlightfoundation.org

The Cutting Edge Catalogue carries many items in the category of health technology, including pH meters, water systems, and books.

Cutting Edge Catalogue
P.O. Box 5034
Southampton, NY 11969
Orders or catalogue: 800-497-9516
Information: 516-287-3813
Fax: 516-287-3112
www.cutcat.com
E-mail: cutcat@i-2000.com

The Living Water Machine
Crystal Clear

Regenesis 2000
Water Purifier and Ionizer
Westbrook Farms Route 209
Westbrookville, NY 12785
Call 845-754-8696 for more information and literature.
www.johnellis.com

Green Power Juicer
Orders: 888-254-7336
Inquiries: 562-940-4241
Fax: 562-940-4240
www.greenpower.com

Vita-Mix Blenders
8615 Usher Road
Cleveland, OH 44138-2199
800-848-2649
www.vita-mix.com

For a wonderful, easy-to-get-started program on sprouting, kits in different sizes, instructions on how to sprout, information on nutritional aspects of different seeds, single seeds, and seed mixes:

Life Sprouts
P.O. Box 150
Hyrum, UT
435-245-3891

There are many organic food distributors, here's one we like:
Whole Foods Market, Inc.
550 Bowie Street
Austin, TX 78703-4644
512-477-4455
512-477-5566 voicemail
512-482-7000 fax
www.wholefoodsmarket.com

Pacific Foods of Oregon
Tualatin, OR 97062
503-692-9666
www.pacificfoods.com

Udo's Choice®
Flora, Inc.
Lyden,WA 98264
800-446-2110
www.udoerasmus.com
www.florainc.com

Arrowhead Mills
(Essential Balance/Omega Nutrition oil)
Vancouver, BC V5L 1P5
800-661-3529
www.omeganutrition.com

Imagine Foods, Inc.
350 Cambridge Ave.
Suite 350
Palo Alto, CA 94306
www.imaginefoods.com

Recommended Reading

The Colon Health Handbook
Robert Gray
Emerald Publishing
Reno, Nevada

Dressed to Kill
Sydney Ross Singer and Soma Grismaijer
Avery Publishing Group
Garden City Park, New York

Earl Mindell's Soy Miracle
Earl Mindell
Simon & Schuster
New York, New York

Enzyme Nutrition
Edward Howell
Avery Publishing Group, Inc.
Wayne, New Jersey

Fats That Heal-Fats That Kill
Udo Erasmus

Alive Books
Burnaby, British Columbia, Canada

The HarperCollins Illustrated Medical Dictionary
HarperCollins
New York, New York

The Healing Power of Chlorophyll from Plant Life
Bernard Jensen
Bernard Jensen Enterprises
Escondido, California

Herbal Nutritional Medications
National Health Research Association
Alpine, Utah

Hidden Killers
Dr. Erik Enby
Semmelweiss-Institut
Steinweg, Germany

A Holistic Protocol for the Immune System
Scott J. Gregory
Tree of Life Publications
Joshua Tree, California

Is This Your Child's World?
Doris J. Rapp, M.D.
Bantam Books
New York, New York

The Juicing Book
Stephen Blaver
Avery Publishing Group, Inc.
Garden City Park, New York

Prescription for Nutritional Healing
J. F. Balch and P. A. Balch
Avery Publishing Group
Garden City Park, New York

Reclaiming Our Health
John Robbins
HJ Kramer, Inc.

P.O. Box 1082
Tiburon, California 94920

Slow Burn
Stu Mittleman
HarperCollins
New York, New York

Touch for Health
John F. Thie, D.C.
DeVorss & Co.
Marina del Rey, California

Wheatgrass Book
Ann Wigmore
Avery Publishing Group, Inc.
Wayne, New Jersey

The Yeast Connection, A Medical Breakthrough
William G. Crook
Professional Books
Jackson, Tennessee

APPENDIX: AN INSIGHTFUL ARTICLE BY DR. ROBERT O. YOUNG

The Cure For ALL Cancers, Heart Disease, Diabetes, Osteoporosis, Lupus, Arthritis, Alzheimer's Has Been Discovered!

Disease, or should we say dis-Ease, and names like Cancer, Heart Disease, Type I and Type II Diabetes, Osteoarthritis, Rheumatoid arthritis, Lupus, Alzheimer's and Osteoporosis are misleading. Not only do they strike fear into our collective hearts, but they misinform patients—and everyone else—about both care and dis-ease prevention and treatment

There is a curious tendency in conventional medicine to take a set of symptoms, string them together, and give the whole thing a name which is then called a disease.

Did I say "curious?" Well yes, but I might add, disconcerting, irresponsible, self-serving, exclusionary and just plain wrong! Once the western medical monopoly names a symptom a disease, they have made a major effort and taken a major step toward baring the door for all other adjunctive and alternative medical professions from getting involved.

I was recently at a compounding pharmacy having my bone mineral density measured to update my health stats. I spotted a poster touting a new drug for osteoarthritis and osteoporosis. It was written by a drug company and it said exactly this:

"Osteoporosis is a dis-ease that causes weak and fragile bones." Then, the poster went on to say that you need a particular drug to counteract this "disease". Yet the language is all backwards.

183

The Cause and Cure for Osteoarthritis, Rheumatoid Arthritis, and Osteoporosis

Osteoarthritis, rheumatoid arthritis and osteoporosis are not diseases that cause weak joints, weak bones, weak tissues and weak organs. For example, Rheumatoid arthritis is the name given to a "diagnosis" of inflammation and degeneration of the joints, tissues and organs. But rheumatoid arthritis does not come from inflamed and degenerative joints. And inflamed and degenerative joints do not come from rheumatoid arthritis. The inflammation and degeneration of the joints are the direct and indirect result of excess dietary and/or metabolic acidity. But then medical doctors follow it up with the fancy diagnosis of rheumatoid arthritis. Just the name sounds scary. The drug companies and their marketing makes it sound like rheumatoid arthritis strikes first, and then you get inflamed and degenerative joints, tissues and organs. The cause and effect is all backwards. And that's how drug companies want people to think about dis-eases and symptoms: first you "get" the dis-ease, and then you are "diagnosed" just in time to take a new drug for the rest of your life. And, of course, you have to keep going back to the doctor for a visit to renew the prescription. But it's all hogwash. There is no such disease as rheumatoid arthritis, osteoarthritis or osteoporosis. It's just a made-up name given to a pattern of acidic lifestyle and diet symptoms that indicates you are over-acid which causes your joints, tissues and organs to become weak, fragile, and inflamed.

The Cause and Cure For High Blood Pressure and High Cholesterol

As another example, when a person follows an unhealthy acidic lifestyle and diet that results in a symptom such as high blood pressure, that symptom is actually being assumed to be a disease all by itself. Then, it is given a disease name. What disease? The dis-ease is, of course, is "hypertension" or "high blood pressure." Doctors throw this phrase around as if it were an actual dis-ease and not merely descriptive of patient physiology.

This may all seem silly, right? But there's actually a very important point to all this. When we look at symptoms and give them disease names, we automatically distort the selection of available treatments for such a dis-ease.

If the dis-ease is, by itself, hypercholesterolemia or high cholesterol, then the cure for the dis-ease must be nothing other than lowering the high cholesterol. And that's how we end up with all these pharmaceuticals treating high cholesterol in order to "prevent" this dis-ease and lower the levels of LDL cholesterol in the human patient. By lowering only the cholesterol, the doctor can rest assured that he is, in fact, treating this "disease," since the definition of this "disease" is hypercholesterolemia or high cholesterol and nothing else.

But there is a fatal flaw in this approach to disease treatment: the symptom is not the cause of the dis-ease. There is another cause, and this deeper cause is routinely ignored by conventional medicine, doctors, drug companies, and even patients. Let's take a closer look at hypertension or high blood pressure.

What actually causes high blood pressure?

Many doctors would say high blood pressure is caused by a specific, measurable interaction between circulating chemicals in the human body. Thus, the ill-behaved chemical compounds are the cause of the high blood pressure, and therefore the solution is to regulate these chemicals. That's exactly what pharmaceuticals do. They attempt to manipulate the chemicals in the body to adjust the symptoms of high blood pressure. Thus, they only treat the symptoms, not the root cause. Or take a look at high cholesterol. The conventional medicine approach says that high cholesterol is caused by a chemical imbalance in the liver which is the organ that produces cholesterol. Thus the treatment for high cholesterol is a prescription drug that inhibits the liver's production of cholesterol (statin drugs). Upon taking these drugs, the high cholesterol (the "disease") is regulated.

But what was causing the liver to overproduce cholesterol in the first place?

That causative factor remains ignored and unaddressed. The base cause or the root cause of high cholesterol, as it turns out, is primarily an over-acidic lifestyle and diet. A person who lives an acidic life is a person who frequently eats foods that are acidic that will inevitably cause the body to go into preservation mode and produce more cholesterol to neutralize the excess acid from that acidic food or drink and thus showing the symptoms of this so-called dis-ease of high cholesterol. Its simple cause and effect.

If you eat the wrong foods and don't exercise, you will produce too much acid which can cause the body to release cholesterol from the liver to bind up that dietary and/or metabolic acid which can be detected and diagnosed by conventional medical procedures.

You see, it is not the cholesterol that is bad. It is the acid-producing food we eat and the lack of exercise that is bad. Reduce the acid-producing foods like beef, chicken, pork, dairy, coffee, tea, soda pop, sports drinks, energy drinks, alcohol, etc. and start exercising every day and you will reduce the protective cholesterol that is saving your life from dietary acids that are not being properly eliminated through the four channels of elimination (urination, perspiration, defecation and respiration).

So, the root cause of all disease, inflammation, degeneration, the increase of blood plasma antibodies or increase blood plasma LDL cholesterol is actually poor lifestyle and food choice, not some bizarre behavior by the liver. If the disease were to be accurately named, then, it would be called "Acidic Lifestyle and Food Choice Dis-Ease", or simply ALFCD. ALFCD would be a far more accurate name that would make sense to most people. If it's an acidic lifestyle and foods choice dis-ease, then it seems that the obvious solution to the dis-ease would be to choose a lifestyle and foods that aren't so acidic or are alkalizing to the blood, tissues and organs.

Of course, that may be a bit of a over-simplification since you have to distinguish between healthy alkaline lifestyles and foods and unhealthy acidic lifestyle and foods. But at least the name ALFCD gives patients a better idea of what's actually going on in their body rather than naming the dis-ease after a symptom such as hypercholesterolemia or rheumatoid arthritis or even cancer.

The symptom is not the dis-ease, but conventional medicine insists on calling the symptom the dis-ease because that way it can treat the symptom and claim success without actually addressing the

186

underlying cause which somehow remains a mystery to modern medicine. But let's move on to some other dis-eases so you get a clearer picture of how this actually works.

The Cause and Cure for Type I and Type II Diabetes

Another dis-ease that's caused by poor lifestyle and acidic food choice is diabetes. Type 1 and Type 2 diabetes is the natural physiological and metabolic result of a person consuming refined carbohydrates and added sugars in large quantities, undigested proteins from beef, chicken, and pork without engaging in regular physical exercise that would compensate for such dietary practices. The name "diabetes" is meaningless to the average person. The disease should be called "Excessive Acid Dis-Ease", or EAD.

If diabetes Type I or Type II were called "Excessive Acid Dis-ease", the solution to it would be rather apparent; simply eliminate ALL sugars, eliminate all animal proteins, eggs, dairy, soft drinks, candy, processed food and be sure to exercise, rest, etc. But, of course, that would be far too simple for the medical community. So the dis-ease must be given a complex name such as Type I or Type II diabetes that puts its solution or cure out of the reach of the average patient.

The Cause and Cure for ALL Cancers

Another dis-ease that is named after its symptom is Cancer. In fact, to this day, most doctors and many patients still believe that Cancer is a physical thing: a tumor. In reality, a tumor is the solution of Cancer, not its cause. A tumor is simply a physical manifestation of bound up acidic cells so they do not spoil other healthy cells. The tumor is the solution to cells damaged by dietary and/or metabolic acids, not the problem but the solution.

The truth is Cancer is not a cell but an acidic poisonous liquid. When a person "has cancer", what they really have is cancerous tissues or "latent tissue acidosis". They are absorbing their own acidic urine. That would be a far better name for ALL forms of Cancer dis-ease: Cancerous Tissue Dis-Ease (CTD) or "Latent Tissue Acidosis" or LTA.

187

If Cancer were actually called "Latent Tissue Acidosis", it would seem ridiculous to try to cure cancer by cutting out tumors through surgery and by destroying the immune or janitorial system with chemotherapy. And yet these are precisely the most popular treatments for Cancer offered by conventional medicine. These treatments do absolutely nothing to support the patients immune system and prevent the build-up of dietary, metabolic, environmental and respiratory acids in the tissues.

That's exactly why most people who undergo chemotherapy or the removal of tumors through surgical procedures end up with more cancerous tumors a few months or a few years later. It's also another reason why survival rates of cancer have barely budged over the last thirty years.

In other words, conventional medicine's treatments for cancer simply don't work!

Bottom line, the main reason treatment doesn't work is that current medical science wrongly perceives Cancer as a cell when in reality Cancer is an acidic poisonous liquid waste product, like lactic acid or uric acid, from what we eat, drink and think.

A good part of this situation stems from the fact that the dis-ease is misnamed "Cancer" to begin with. But it isn't a tumor and it certainly isn't a dis-ease caused by having an immune system which is too strong and that needs to be destroyed through chemotherapy. It is simply "latent tissue acidosis". And if it were called "latent tissue acidosis dis-ease" or "urine-in-the-tissues dis-ease", the effective treatment for cancer would be apparent.

There are many other dis-eases that are given misleading names by western medicine. But if you look around the world and take a look at how dis-eases are named elsewhere, you will find many countries have dis-ease names that actually make sense.

For example, in Chinese medicine, Alzheimer's dis-ease is given a name that means, when translated, "feeble mind disease". In Chinese medicine, the name of the dis-ease more accurately describes the actual cause of the dis-ease which is caused by acids or urine on the brain, whereas in western medicine, the name of the dis-ease seems to be intended to obscure the root cause of the dis-ease, thereby making all dis-eases sound far more complex and mysterious than they really are. This is one way in which medical and some alternative doctors and practitioners of western medicine keep medical treatments out of the reach of the average person. Because, good Heavens, they sure don't want people thinking for themselves about the true causes of disease!

By creating a whole new vocabulary for medical conditions, medical doctors can speak their own secret language and make sure that people who aren't schooled in medicine don't understand what they're saying. That's a shame, because the treatments and cures for virtually all acute and chronic dis-eases are actually quite simple and can be described in plain language: They include making different alkaline food choices, getting more natural sunlight, drinking more alkaline water, engaging in regular physical exercise, avoiding specific acidic foods, supplementing our diet with green foods and green drinks, alkalizing nutritional supplements, and so on.

Western medicine prefers to describe dis-eases in terms of chemistry. When you're depressed, you aren't suffering from a lack of natural sunlight; you are suffering from a "brain chemistry imbalance" that can only be regulated, they claim, by ingesting toxic chemicals to alter your brain chemistry.

When your bones are brittle, it's not "acidic brittle bones dis-ease"; it's called osteoporosis, something that sounds very technical and complicated. Or when your joints are inflamed and degenerating, it's not called "acidic connective tissue disease" or "I absorb my own urine disease", it's called rheumatoid arthritis. And to treat all of these acidic conditions, western doctors and physicians will give you prescriptions for expensive drugs that somehow claim to make your bones less brittle or use acidic steroids to make your joints less inflamed. But in fact, the real treatment for these acidic symptomologies can be described in plain language once again: regular physical exercise, vitamin D supplementation, mineral supplements that include sodium, magnesium and strontium, natural sunlight, and avoidance of acidic foods such as soft drinks, white flour, added sugars, dairy products, that increases uric acid, carbonic acid, lactose and lactic acid in the tissues and of course all animal proteins which release the poisonous acids of nitric, uric, sulphuric and phosphoric acid into the blood and

189

connective tissues. All of these acids, if not eliminated through the four channels of elimination can only lead to one thing - acidic chronic inflammation and then degeneration of the connective tissues, organs and glands.

In fact, virtually every dis-ease that is prominent in modern society—diabetes, heart disease, cancer, osteoarthritis, rheumatoid arthritis, osteoporosis, clinical depression, irritable bowel syndrome, Parkinson's, Lupus, Alzheimer's, and so on—can be easily described in plain language without using complex terms at all.

These dis-eases are simply misnamed. And I believe that they are intentionally misnamed to put the jargon out of reach of everyday people. As a result, there's a great deal of arrogance in the language of western medicine. This arrogance furthers the language of separation. Separation never results in healing.

> **Healing (literally meaning to *make whole* {Oxford English Dictionary}) is the process of restoring health to an unbalanced/ diseased/damaged organism.**

In order to effect healing, we must bring together the language of healers and patients using plain language that real people understand and upon which real people can act. We need to start describing dis-eases in terms of their root causes, not in terms of their arcane, biochemical actions. When someone suffers from seasonal affective disorder or clinical depression, for example, let's call it what it is: "Sunlight Deficiency Disorder". To treat it, the person simply needs to get more sunlight. This isn't rocket science, it's not complex, and it doesn't require a prescription from Big Bucks Pharma.

If someone is suffering from rheumatoid arthritis, let's get realistic about the words we use to describe the condition: it's really "Acidic Connective Joint and Tissue Dis-ease". And it should be treated with things that will reduce the acids that cause inflammation and degeneration, such as nutrition, physical exercise and avoidance of acidic foods and drinks that strip away bone mass, cause inflammation and degeneration from the human body to neutralize the excess acids in the blood and then joints, tissues, organs and glands.

All of this information, of course, is rather shocking to old-school

190

medical doctors and practitioners of western medicine. And unfortunately, the bigger their egos and insecurity, the more they dislike the idea of naming dis-eases in plain language that patients can actually comprehend.

That's because if the simple truths about dis-eases and their causes were known, health would be more readily available to everyday people, and that would lessen the importance of physicians and medical researchers. There's a great deal of ego invested in the medical community, and they sure don't want to make sound health attainable to the average person without their expert acidic advice.

Many medical doctors want to serve as the translators of "truth" and will balk at any attempts to educate the public to either practice medicine on their own. But in reality, health (and a connection with spirit) is attainable by every single person that resides on planet earth.

Health is easy, it is straightforward, it is direct and, for the most part, it is available free of charge. A personal connection with our Creator is the same if we ask humbly in prayer for a relationship with Him, and guidance.

Don't believe the names of dis-eases given to you by your medical doctor. Those names are designed to obscure, not to inform. They are designed to separate you from self-healing, not to put you in touch with your own inner healer. And thus, they are nothing more than bad medicine masquerading as modern medical practice.

In conclusion, it is acid that causes an allergic reaction NOT exercise. It is dietary, metabolic, environmental and respiratory acids that KILL - NOT EXERCISE. If you do not make time to exercise and remove the acids that cause ALL sickness and disease you will need to make time to DIE!

The Cure for ALL human and animal sickness and disease, including the BIG three, Cancer, Diabetes and Heart Disease is found in its 'Prevention' not in its 'Cure'.

To learn more about an alkalizing lifestyle and diet read the pH Miracle 1 and 2, The pH Miracle for Diabetes, The pH Miracle for Weight Loss and The pH Miracle for Cancer by Dr. Robert O. Young or go to our website at: www.phmiracle.com

REFERENCES

2004 *Physicians' Desk Reference*, 58th ed. Stamford: Thomson Health Care, Inc.; 2003.

Adetumbi, M. A., Javor, C. F., and Lau, B. H. S. Anti-Candida activity of garlic-effect on macromolecular synthesis. Presented at the American Society for Microbiology, Loma Linda University, 1985.

Alberts, B., et al., eds. *Molecular Biology of the Cell*, 2d ed. New York: Garland Publishing, Inc., 1989.

Aleksandrowixz, J., and Smyk, B. Mycotoxins and their role in oncogenesis with special reference to blood diseases. *Polish Medical Science Historical Bulletin*, 1971; 24: 25-30.

Alexander, J. G. Allergy in the gastrointestinal tract. *Lancet*, 1975; 2: 1264.

Alpert, M. E., Hutt, M. S. R., Wogan, G. N., and Davidson, C. S. Association between aflatoxin content and hepatoma frequency in Uganda. *Cancer*, 1971; 28: 253.

Anderson, M.E., Luo, J.L. Glutathione therapy: from prodrugs to genes. *Semin Liver Dis.*, 1998; 18:415-424.

Aso, H., et al. Induction of interferon and activation of NK cells and macrophages in mice by oral administration of Ge-132, an organic germanium compound. *Journal of Microbiology and Immunology*, 1985; 29(1): 65-74.

Avdic, E., "Bicarbonate versus acetate hemodialysis: effects on the acid-base status" (Med Arh 2001; 55(4):231-3).

Aw, T.W., Wierzbicka G., Jones D.P. Oral glutathione increases tissue glutathione in vivo. *Chemico-biological Interactions*, 1991; 80:89-97.

Bains, J.S., Shaw, C.A. Neurodegenerative disorders in humans: the role of glutathione in oxidative stress-mediated neuronal death. *Brain Research Reviews*, 1997; 25:335-358.

Bakhir, V. *Electrochemical Activation*, 2 vol. All-Russian Institute for Medical Engineering, Moscow, 1992.

Barker, N. et al. Identification of stem cells in small intestine and colon by marker gene Lgr5. *Nature*, 449, 1003-7 (25 October 2007).

Batmanghelidj, F. *Your Body's Many Cries for Water*. Global Health Solutions, Falls Church, VA, 1992.

Béchamp, Pierre Jacques Antoine. *The Blood and Its Third Anatomical Element* (Montague R. Leverson, translator). London: John Ouseley Limited, 1912.

Becker, Robert O., M.D., and Selden, Gary. *The Body Electric. Electromagnetism and the Foundation of Life*. New York: Quill/William Morrow, 1985.

Bertz, A., et al. Modulation by cytokines of leukocyte endothelial cell interactions. Implications for thrombosis. *Biorheology*, 1990; 27: 455.

Bick, R. L. Disseminated intravascular coagulation. *Hematology/Oncology Clinics of North America*, 1993; 6: 1259.

Bird, Christopher. *Gaston Naessens*. Tiburon, Calif.: H. J. Kramer, Inc., 1991.

_____. *The Galileo of the Microscope*. St. Lambert, Quebec, Canada: Les Presses de l'Université de la Personne, Inc., 1990.

_____. To Be or Not to Be? A paper presented in an address to L'Orthobiologie Smatidienne Symposium 1991, Sherbrooke, Quebec, hosted by Gaston Naessens.

Blank, F. O., Chin, G., Just, B., et al. Carcinogens from fungi pathogenic for man. *Cancer Research*, 1968; 28: 2276.

Bleker, Dr. Maria. *Blood Examination in Darkfield According to Professor Dr. Günther Enderlein*. Gesamtherstellung, Germany: Semmelweis-Verlag, 1993.

Boeing, H., Schlehofer, B., Blettner, M., Wahrendorf, J. Dietary carcinogens and the risk for glioma and meningioma in Germany. *International Journal of Cancer*, 1993; 53(4): 561-65.

Bohn T, Walczyk S, Leisibach S, Hurrell RF. Chlorophyll-bound magnesium in commonly consumed vegetables and fruits:

relevance to magnesium nutrition. *The Journal of Food Science*, 2004; 69(9): S347-S350.

Bolton, S., and Null, G. The medical uses of garlic: Fact and fiction. *American Pharmacy*, August 1982.

Borok Z, Buhl R, Grimes GJ, et al. Effect of glutathione aerosol on oxidant-antiox- dant imbalance in ideopathic pulmonary fi brosis. *Lancet*. 1991; 338:215-216.

Bowers W.F. Chlorophyll in wound healing and suppurative disease. *Journal of the American Society of Plastic Surgeons*, 1947;73:37-50.

Bowie, E. J., et al. The clinical pathology of intravascular coagulation. *Bibliotheca Haematologica*, 1983; 49: 217.

Bredbacka, S., et al. Laboratory methods for detecting disseminated intravascular coagulation (DIC): New aspects. *Acta Anaesthesiologica Scandinavica*, 1993; 37: 125.

Breen, F. A., et al. Ethanol gelation: A rapid screening test for intravascular coagulation. *Annals of Internal Medicine*, 1970; 69: 1197.

Breinholt, V., Hendricks, J., Pereira, C., Arbogast, D., Bailey, G. Dietary chlorophyllin is a potent inhibitor of aflatoxin B1 hepatocarcinogenesis in rainbow trout. *Cancer Research*, 1995;55(1):57-62.

Breinholt, V., Schimerlik, M., Dashwood, R., Bailey, G. Mechanisms of chlorophyllin anticarcinogenesis against aflatoxin B1: complex formation with the carcinogen. *Chemical Research in Toxicology*, 1995;8(4):506-514.

Broquist, H.P. Buthionine sulfoximine, an experimental tool to induce glutathionine deficiency: elucidation of glutathionine and ascorbate in their role as antioxidants. *Nutrition Review*, 1992; 50:110-111.

Brown, L.A., Bai, C., Jones, D.P. Glutathione protection in alveolar type II cells from fetal and neonatal rabbits. *American Journal of Physiology*, 1992; 262:L305-L312.

Burkitt, D. Some disease characteristics of modern Western civilization. *British Medical Journal*, 1973; 1: 274.

Carp, H., et al. In vitro suppression of serum elastase-inhibitory capacity by ROTS genera ted by phagocytosing polymorphonuclear leukocytes. *Journal of Clinical Investigation*, 1979; 63: 793.

Carpenter, E.B. Clinical experiences with chlorophyll preparations. *American Journal of Surgery*, 1949; 77: 167-171.

Cascinu, S., Cordella, L., Del Ferro, E., et al. Neuroprotective effect of reduced glutathione on cisplatin-based chemotherapy in advanced gastric cancer: a randomized double-blind placebo-controlled study. *Journal of Clinical Oncology*, 1995; 13:26-32.

Chandler, W. L., et al. Evaluation of a new dynamic viscometer for measuring the viscosity of whole blood and plasma. *Clinical Chemistry*, 1986; 32: 505.

Chen, F., Cole, P., Mi, Z., Xing, L. Y. Corn and wheat-flour consumption and mortality from esophageal cancer in Shanxi, China. *International Journal of Cancer*, 1993; 4(2): 163-69.

Chernomorsky, S.A., Segelman, A.B. Biological activities of chlorophyll derivatives. *New Jersey Medicine*, 1988; 85(8):669-673.

Cheung, P-Y, Wang, W., Schulz, R. Glutathione protects against ischemiaperfusion injury by detoxifying peroxynitrite. *Journal of Molecular and Cellular Cardiology*, 2000; 32:1669-1678.

Chimploy, K., Diaz, G.D., Li, Q., et al. *International Journal of Cancer*, 2009; in press.

Cho, T. H., et al. Effects of *Escherichia coli* toxin on structure and permeability of myocardial capillaries. Acta *Pathologica Japonica*, 1991; 41: 12.

Christiansen, S.B., Byel, S.R., Stromsted, H., Stenderup, J.K., Eickhoff, J.H. [Can chlorophyll reduce fecal odor in colostomy patients?]. *Ugeskr Laeger*, 1989; 151(27): 1753-1754.

Colucci, M., et al. Cultured human endothelial cells: An in vitro model of vascular injury. *Journal of Clinical Investigation*, 1983; 71: 1893.

Cooper, L. A., and Gadd, G. M. Differentiation and melanin production in hyaline and pigmented strains of *Microdochium bolleyi*. In Constantini, A. V., Weiland, H., Qvick, Lars I. *The Fungal/Mycotoxin Etiology of Human Disease*, Vol. 2. Freiburg, Germany: Johann Friedrich Oberlin Verlag, 1994.

Cope, Freeman W. Evidence from activation energies for superconductive tunneling in biological systems at physiological temperatures. *Physiological Chemistry and Physics*, 1971; 3: 403-10.

Costantini, A. V., Weiland, H., Qvick, Lars I. *The Fungal/Mycotoxin Etiology of Human Disease*, Volumes 1 and 2. Freiburg, Germany: Johann Friedrich Oberlin Verlag, 1994.

Cusumano, V. Aflatoxin in patients with lung cancer. *Oncology*, 1991; 48: 194-95.

Dashwood, R., Yamane S, Larsen R. Study of the forces of stabilizing complexes between chlorophylls and heterocyclic amine mutagens. Environ Mol Mutagen. 1996;27(3): 211-218.

Dashwood, R.H., Breinholt, V., Bailey, G.S. Chemopreventive properties of chlorophyllin: inhibition of aflatoxin B1 (AFB1)-DNA binding in vivo and anti-mutagenic activity against AFB1 and two heterocyclic amines in the Salmonella mutagenicity assay. *Carcinogenesis*, 1991; 12(5):939-942.

Dashwood R.H. The importance of using pure chemicals in (anti) mutagenicity studies: chlorophyllin as a case in point. Mutat Res. 1997; 381(2):283-286.

Dawson-Huges, B. "Treatment with Potassium Bicarbonate Lowers Calcium Excretion and Bone Resorption in Older Men and Women," *The Journal of Clinical Endocrinology & Metabolism*, Vol. 94, No. 1 96-102.

De Mattia, G., Bravi, M.C., Laurenti, O., et al. Influence of reduced glutathione infusion on glucose metabolism in patients with non-insulin-dependent diabetes mellitus. *Metabolism*, 1998; 47:993-997.

Dement'eva, I.I. "Calculation of the dose of sodium bicarbonate in the treatment of metabolic acidosis in surgery with (and) deep hypothermic circulatory arrest" (Anesteziol Reanimatol 1997 Sep-Oct; 5:42-4).

Dickens, L. *Carcinogenesis: A Broad Critique.* Baltimore: Williams & Wilkins, 1967.

Dickens, R., and Jones, H. E. H. Further studies on the carcinogenic action of patulin-induced mammary adenomas and local sarcomas or fibrosarcomas in mice and rats. *British Journal of Cancer*, 1965; 19: 392.

Dingley, K.H., Ubick, E.A., Chiarappa-Zucca, M.L., et al. Effect of dietary constituents with chemopreventive potential on adduct formation of a low dose of the heterocyclic amines PhIP and IQ and phase II hepatic enzymes. *Nutrition and Cancer*, 2003; 46(2): 212-221.

Duke, Don, M. S. Materials rich in monoatomic elements [report on personal research]. Phoenix, Ariz., 1995.

Egner, P.A., Munoz, A., Kensler, T.W. Chemoprevention with chlorophyllin in individuals exposed to dietary aflatoxin. *Mutat Res.* 2003;523-524:209-216.

Egner, P.A., Stansbury, K.H., Snyder, E.P., Rogers, M.E., Hintz, P.A., Kensler, T.W. Identification and characterization of chlorine (4) ethyl ester in sera of individuals participating in the chlorophyllin chemoprevention trial. *Chemical Research in Toxicology*, 2000; 13(9): 900-906.

Egner, P.A., Wang, J.B., Zhu, Y.R., et al. Chlorophyllin intervention reduces aflatoxin-DNA adducts in individuals at high risk for liver cancer. *Proceedings of the National Academy of Sciences*, 2001; 98(25):14601-14606.

El-Osta, Assam et al. "Transient high glucose causes persistent epigenetic changes and altered gene expression during subsequent normoglycemia." *Journal of Experimental Medicine*, Vol. 205, No. 10, 2409-2417.

Encyclopedia of Chemical Technology. New York: John Wiley and Sons, 1983.

Enderlein, Prof. Dr. Günther. Akmon, Volume I, Books 1 and 2. Hamburg, Germany: Ibica-Verlag, 1957.

_____. *Bakterien Cyclogenie.* Hamburg, Germany: Ibica-Verlag, 1925.

197

Enomoto, M. Carcinogenicity of mycotoxins. *In Toxicology, Biochemistry and Pathology of Mycotoxins* (Uraguchi, K., and Yamazaki, M., eds.). New York: John Wiley & Son, 1978.

Erickson, B.L. and Wullaert, R.A. Expanding a new scientific view of the functional properties of water.

_____. *Proceedings of the Functional Water Symposiums*, (1994-2000), Tokyo, Japan.

Exner, R., Wessner, B., Manhart, N., Roth, E. Therapeutic potential of glutathione. *Wiener Klinische Wochenschrift*, 2000; 112: 610-616.

Favilli, F., Marraccini, P., Iantomasi, T., Vincenzini, M.T. Effect of orally administered glutathione levels in osme organs of rats: role of specifi c transporters. *British Journal of Nutrition*, 1997; 78: 293-300.

Feriani, M., Randomized long-term evaluation of bicarbonate-buffered CAPD solution. *Kidney International*, 1998; Nov; 54(5):1731-8.

Fernandes, G. Effect of Electrolyzed Water Intake on Lifespan of Autoimmune Disease Prone Mice. FASEB *Journal*, 12 (1998); A794.

Fink-Gemmels, J. The significance of mycotoxin assimilation of meat animals. *Deutsche Tierärztliche Wochenschift*, 1989; 96(7): 360-63.

Flagg, E.W., Coates, R.J., Eley, J.W., et al. Dietary glutathione intake in humans and the relationship between intake and plasma total glutathionine level. *Nutrition and Cancer*, 1994; 21:33-46.

Franceschi, E. A. Meat, poultry, cooked ham, salami, sausages, cheese, butter and oil-related thyroid cancer. *International Journal of Cancer*, 1993; 53(4): 561-65.

Fungalbionics Convention: The Fungal/Mycotoxin Etiology of Chronic and Degenerative Disease. Metro Toronto Convention Centre, September 30, 1994.

Furukawa, T., Meydani, S.N., Blumberg, J.B. Reversal of age-associated decline in immune responsiveness by dietary glutathione supplementation in mice. *Mechanisms of Ageing and Development*, 1987; 38:107-117.

Gamba, G., Bicarbonate therapy in severe diabetic ketoacidosis. A double blind, randomized, placebo controlled trial. *Revista de Investigacion Clinica*, 1991, Jul-Sep; 43(3):234-8). Miyares Gomez A. in Diabetic ketoacidosis in childhood: the fi rst day of treatment. *Anales de Pediatria*, 1989 Apr; 30(4): 279-83).

Ghadirian, P. Thermal irritation and esophageal cancer in northern Iran. *Cancer*, 1987; 60(8): 1909-14.

Giovannucci, E., Rimm, E. B., Colditz, G. A., Stampfer, M. J., Ascherio, A., Chute, C. C., and Willett, W. C. A prospective study of mycotoxins and risk of prostate cancer. *Journal of the National Cancer Institute*, 1993; 85(19): 1538-40.

Gogel, H.K., Tandberg, D., Strickland, R.G.. Substances that interfere with guaiac card tests: implications for gastric aspirate testing. *American Journal of Emergency Medicine*, 1989;7(5):474-480.

Griffith, O.W. Biologic and pharmacologic regulation of mammalian glutathione synthesis. *Free Radical Biology & Medicine*, 1999; 27:922-935.

Grimstad, I. A., et al. Thromboplastin release, but not content, correlates with spontaneous metastasis of cancer cells. *International Journal of Cancer*, 1988; 41: 427.

Gunji, Y., et al. Role of fi brin coagulation in protection of murine tumor cells from destruction by cytotoxic cells. *Cancer Research*, 1988; 48: 5216. Hagen, T.M., Jones, D.P. Transepithelial transport of glutathione in vascularly perfused small intestine of rat. *American Journal of Physiology*, 1987; 252(5 Pt 1): G607-G613.

Hagen, T.M., Wierzbicka, G.T., Sillau, A.H., et al. Bioavailability of dietary glutathione: effect on plasma concentration. *American Journal of Physiology*, 1990; 259(4 Pt 1):G524-G529.

Hamilton, P. J., et al. Disseminated intravascular coagulation: A review. *Journal of Clinical Pathology*, 1978; 31: 609.

Hanaoka, K. Antioxidant Effects of Reduced Water Produced by Electrolysis of Sodium Chloride Solutions (to be published in *Journal of Applied Electrochemistry*, 2001).

Hay, E. D., ed. *Cell Biology of Extracellular Matrix*. New York: Plenum Press, 1981.

Hayes, J.D., McLellan, L.I. Glutathione and glutathione-dependent enzymes represent a co-ordinately regulated defence against oxidative stress. *Free Radical Research*, 1999; 31:273-300.

Hayes, J.D., Strange, R.C. Glutathione S-transferase polymorphisms and their biological consequences. *Pharmacology*, 2000; 61:154-166.

Heinicke, R. M. The pharmacologically active ingredient of noni [a paper]. University of Hawaii, January 1996.

Hendler, S.S., Rorvik D.R., eds. *PDR for Nutritional Supplements.* 2nd ed. Montvale: Physicians' Desk Reference, Inc; 2008.

Hercbergs, A., Brok-Simoni, F., Holtzman, F., et al. Erythrocyte glutathione and tumor response to chemotherapy. *Lancet*, 1992; 339:1074-1076.

Hertog, M. G., Feskens, E. J., Hollmati, P. C., Katan, M. B., and Kromhout,

D. Dietary antioxidants and risk of coronary disease. *Lancet*, 1993; 342: 32-34.

Hills, Christopher. *Nuclear Evolution.* Boulder Creek, Calif.: University of the Trees Press, 1977.

Holroyd, K.J., Buhl, R., Borok, Z., et al. Correction of glutathione defi ciency in the lower respiratory tract of HIV seropositive individuals by glutathione aerosol treatment. *Thorax*, 1993; 48:985-989.

Hu, T., et al. Synthesis of tissue factor messenger RNA and procoagulant activity in breast cancer cells in response to serum stimulation. *Thrombosis Research*, 1993; 72: 155.

Hudson, David. Alchemical research: DNA alteration and the rediscovery of the light of life. Yelm, Wash.: *Leading Edge Research*; Article 79, February 1995.

Hume, E. Douglas. *Béchamp or Pasteur? A Lost Chapter in the History of Biology*, 1st ed. Ashingdon, Rochford, Essex, England: The C. W. Daniel Company, 1923; 2d. ed. (London: C. W. Daniel Company, 1932) reprinted by Health Research: Pomeroy, Wash., 1989.

Hunder, G., Schumann, K., Strugala, G., Gropp, J., Fichtl, B., and Forth, W. Influence of subchronic exposure to low dietary deoxynivalenol, a trichothecene mycotoxin, on intestinal absorption of nutrients in mice. *Food Chemistry Toxicology*, 1991; 29(12): 809-14.

Hwang, C., Sinskey, A.J., Lodish, H.F. Oxidized redox state of glutathione in the endoplasmic reticulum. *Science*. 1992; 257:1496-1502.

Ingram, D. M., Nottage, E., and Roberts, T. The role *of Saccharomyces cerevisiae*-baker's, or brewer's, yeast-in the development of breast cancer: A case-control study of patients with breast cancer, benign epithelial hyperplasia and fibrocystic disease of the breast. *British Journal of Cancer*, 1991; 64(1): 187-91.

Iwata, K., ed. *Yeasts and Yeast-Like Micro-Organisms in Medical Science*. Tokyo: University of Tokyo Press, 1976.

Janaky, R., Ogita, K., Pasqualotta, B.A., et al. Glutathione and signal transduction in the mammalian CNS. Journal of Neurochemistry, 1999; 73:889-902.

Jones, T. W. Observations on some points in the anatomy, physiology, and pathology of the blood. *British Foreign Medical Review*, 1842; 14: 585.

Jonsyn, Lahai. Aspergillus/aflatoxin contamination of dried fi sh. *International Journal of Cancer*, 1991; 4(1): 8-11.

Kalokerinos, A., and Dettman, G. *Second Thoughts About Disease: A Controversy and Béchamp Revisited*. Warburton, Victoria, Australia: Biological Research Institute [booklet published from an article in *Journal of the International Academy of Preventive Medicine*, July 1977; 4(1): 18].

Kamat, J.P., Boloor, K.K., Devasagayam, T.P. Chlorophyllin as an effective antioxidant against membrane damage in vitro and ex vivo. *Biochimica et Biophysica Acta*, 2000;1487(2-3):113-127.

Kensler, T.W., Groopman, J.D., Roebuck, B.D. Use of aflatoxin adducts as intermediate endpoints to assess the efficacy of chemopreventive interventions in animals and man. *Mutation Research*, 1998; 402(1-2):165-172.

Kephart, J.C. Chlorophyll derivatives-their chemistry, commercial preparation, and uses. *Economic Botany*, 1955;9:3-38.

Keys, A. The role of the diet in human atherosclerosis and its complications. In *Atherosclerosis and Its Origin* (Sandler, M., and Bourne, G. H., eds.). New York and London: Academic Press, 1963.

Kikuchi, S., Okamoto, N., Suzuki, T., Kawahara, S., Nagai, H., Sakiyama, T., Wada, O., and Inaba, Y. A case-control study of breast cancer/mammary cyst and dietary, drinking or smoking habits in Japan. *Japanese Journal of Cancer Clinics*, 1990; 24: 365-69.

Kleiner, S. Water: An Essential but Overlooked Nutrient, *Journal of the American Dietetic Association*, 99 (1999) 200.

Kono, S., Imanishi, K., Shinchi, K., Yanai, F. Relationship of diet to small and large adenomas of the sigmoid colon. *Japan Journal of Cancer Research*, 1993; 84(1): 9-13.

Kumar, S.S., Devasagayam, T.P., Bhushan, B., Verma, N.C. Scavenging of reactive oxygen species by chlorophyllin: an ESR study. *Free Radical Research*, 2001; 35(5):563-574.

Kumar, S.S., Shankar, B., Sainis, K.B. Effect of chlorophyllin against oxidative stress in splenic lymphocytes in vitro and in vivo. *Biochimica et Biophysica Acta*, 2004; 1672(2):100-111.

Kumon, K. What is Functional Water? *Artificial Organs*, 21 (1997) 2.

Kwon-Chung, K. J., and Bennet, John E. *Medical Mycology*. Malvern, Penn.: Lea and Febiger, 1992.

La Vecchia, C., Decarli, A., Negri, E., Parazzini, F., Gentile, A., Cecchetti, G., Fasoli, M., and Franceschi, S. Dietary factors and the risk of epithelial ovarian cancer. *Journal of the National Cancer Institute*, 1987; 79(4): 663-69.

La Vecchia, C., Negri, E., Decarli, A., D'Avanzo, B., and Franceschi, S. A case-control study of diet and gastric cancer in northern Italy. *International Journal of Cancer*, 1987; 40(4): 484-89.

Lancaster, M. C., Jenkins, F. P., and Philp, J. M. C. L. Toxicity associated with certain samples of broken or ground nuts. *Nature*, 1961; 192: 1095-96.

Larsson, S.C., Orsini, N. and Wolk, A. Processed Meat Consumption and Stomach Cancer Risk: A Meta-Analysis, *Journal of the National Cancer Institute*, August 2, 2006; 98(15): 1078-1087.

Lash, L.H., Hagen, T.M., Jones, D.P. Exogenous glutathione protects intestinal epithelial cells from oxidative injury. *Proceedings of the National Academy of Sciences*, 1986; 83:4641-4645.

Lenzi, A., Culasso, F., Gandini, L., et al. Placebo-controlled, double-blind, cross-over trial of glutathione therapy in male infertility. *Human Reproduction*, 1993; 8:1657-1662.

Lenzi, A., Picardo, M., Gandini, L., et al. Glutathione treatment of dyspermia: effect on the lipoperoxidation process. *Human Reproduction*, 1994; 9:2044-2050.

Levi, F., Franceschi, S., Negri, E., and La Vecchia, C. Dietary factors and the risk of endometrial cancer. *Cancer*, 1993; 71(11): 3575-81.

Levy, M. M. An evidence-based evaluation of the use of sodium bicarbonate during cardiopulmonary resuscitation. *Critical Care Clinic*, Jul, 1998; 14(3):457-83). Vukmir, R.B., Sodium bicarbonate in cardiac arrest: a reappraisal *American Journal of Emergency Medicine*, 1996 Mar; 14(2):192-206. Bar-Joseph, G., Clinical use of sodium bicarbonate during cardiopulmonary resuscitation-is it used sensibly? (*Resuscitation*, Jul, 2002; 54(1):47-55).

Linderfelser, L. A., Lillehoj, E. B., and Burnmeister, H. R. Aflatoxin and trichothecene toxins: Skin tumor induction and synergistic acute toxicity in white mice. *Journal of the National Cancer Institute*, 1974; 52: 113.

Livingston-Wheeler, Virginia, MD *The Conquest of Cancer.* New York: Franklin Watts, 1984.

Loguercio, C, Di Pierro, M. The role of glutathione in the gastrointestinal tract: a review. *Italian Journal of Gastroenterology and Hepatology*, 1999; 31:401-407.

Longenecker, Gesina L., PhD *How Drugs Work.* Emeryville, Calif.: Ziff-Davis Press, 1994.

Lorber, A., et al. Clinical application of heavy metal complexing of N-actyl cysteine. *Journal of Clinical Pharmacology*, 1973; 13: 332-36.

Lynes, Barry. *The Cancer Cure That Worked! Fifty Years of Suppression.* Queensville, Ontario, Canada: Marcus Books, 1987.

Lyons J., Rauh-Pfeiffer A., Yu Y.M., et al. Blood glutathione synthesis rates in healthy adults receiving a sulfur amino acid-free diet. *Proceedings of the National Academy of Sciences,* 2000; 97:5071-5076.

Mackman, et al. Lipopolysaccharides-mediated transcriptional activation of the human tissue factor gene in THP-1 monocytic cells requires both activator protein 1 and nuclear factor kappa B binding sites. *Journal of Experimental Medicine,* 1991; 174: 1517.

Maier-Kopf, P. Complexes of metals other than platinum as anti-tumor agents. *Journal of Clinical Pharmacology,* 1994; 47: 1-16.

Margolis, J. The interrelationship of coagulation of plasma and release of peptides. *Annals of the New York Academy of Sciences,* 1963; 104: 133.

Margulis, Lynn, and Sagan, Dorion. *Micro-Cosmos.* New York: Summit Books, 1986.

Mariano, F. Insufficient correction of blood bicarbonate levels in biguanide lactic acidosis treated with CVVH and bicarbonate replacement fluids. *Minerva Urologica e nefrologica,* Sept. 1997; 49(3): 133-6.

Martensson, J., Jain, A., Meister A. Glutathione is required for intestinal function. *Proceedings of the National Academy of Sciences,* 1990; 87:1715-1719.

Matthews, C.K., van Holde, K.E. *Biochemistry.* 2nd ed. Menlo Park: The Benjamin/Cummings Publishing Company; 1996.

Mattman, Lida H. *Cell Wall Deficient Forms-Stealth Pathogens.* Cleveland: CRC Press, 1974.

Meister A. On the antioxidant effects of ascorbic acid and glutathionine. *Biochemical Pharmacology,* 1992; 44:1905-1915.

Miles, M. R., Olsen, L., and Rogers, A. Recurrent vaginal candidiasis; importance of an intestinal reservoir. *Journal of the American Medical Association,* 1977; 238: 1836-37.

Morrison, D. C., et al. The effects of bacterial endotoxins on host mediation systems. *American Journal of Pathology*, 1978; 93: 526.

Motola, Lynne. Hidden in plain sight, the meaning of "grass" in Hebrew. *Western Wheatgrass Journal*, January-March 1995; 2(1): 3-4.

Mueller, H. E., et al. Increase of microbial neuraminidase activity by the hydrogen peroxide concentration. *Experientia*, 1972; 23: 397.

Muller-Berghaus, G., et al. The role of granulocytes in the activation of intravascular coagulation and the precipitation of soluble fibrin by endotoxin. *Blood*, 1975; 45: 631.

Murphy, M.E., Scholich, H., Sies, H. Protection by glutathione and other thiol compounds against the loss of protein thiols and tocopherol homologs during microsomal lipid peroxidation. *European Journal of Biochemistry*, 1992; 210:139-146.

Nachman, R. L., et al. Detection of intravascular coagulation by a serialdilution protamine sulfate test. *Annals of Internal Medicine*, 1971; 75: 895.

_____. Hypercoagulable states. *Annals of Internal Medicine*, 1993; 119: 819.

Nagasawa, H.T., Cohen, J.F., Holleschau, A.M., Rathbun, W.B. Augmentation of human and rat lenticular glutathione in vitro by prodrugs of gamma-Lglutamyl-L-cysteine. *Journal of Medicinal Chemistry*, 1996; 39:1676-1681.

Neuhauser, I., and Gustus, E. L. Successful treatment of intestinal moniliasis with fatty acid resin complex. *Archives of Internal Medicine*, 1954; 93: 53-60.

New Frontier Newsletter. Salt Lake City: New Frontiers, Inc., November 1994.

Norell, S. E., Ahlbom, A., Erwald, R., Jacobson, G., Lindberg-Navier, I., Olin, R., Tornberg, B., and Wiechel, K. L. Diet and pancreatic cancer: A casecontrol study. *American Journal of Epidemiology*, 1986; 124(6): 894-902.

Novi, A.M. Regression of aflatoxin B1-induced hepatocellular carcinomas by reduced glutathione. *Science*, 1981; 212: 541-542.

Ohinataab, Y., Yamasobac, T., Schachta, J., Millera, J.M. Glutathione limits noise-induced hearing loss. *Hearing Research*, 2000; 146:28-34.

Olson, Rick. *Ionized Alkaline Water Using Platinum Electrolysis, Micro-Water and Coral Calcium* [proprietary marketing pamphlet for Coral Calcium]. Olympia, Wash.: Vitality Press and Product Information, September 1995.

Orner, G.A., Roebuck, B.D., Dashwood, R.H., Bailey, G.S. Post-initiation chlorophyllin exposure does not modulate aflatoxin-induced foci in the liver and colon of rats. *Journal of Carcinogenesis*, 2006; 5:6.

Palamara, A.T., Perno, C-F, Ciriolo, M.R., et al. Evidence for antiviral activity of glutathione: in vitro inhibition of herpes simplex virus type 1 replication. *Antiviral Research*, 1995; 27:237-253.

Paolisso, G., Giugliano, D., Pizza, G., et al. Glutathione infusion potentiates glucose-induced insulin secretion in aged patients with impaired glucose tolerance. *Diabetes Care*, 1992; 15:1-7.

Park, K.K., Park, J.H., Jung, Y.J., Chung, W.Y. Inhibitory effects of chlorophyllin, hemin and tetrakis(4-benzoic acid)porphyrin on oxidative DNA damage and mouse skin inflammation induced by 12-O-tetradecanoylphorbol-13-acetate as a possible anti-tumor promoting mechanism. *Mutation Research*, 2003; 542(1-2):89-97

Pasquale, A. D., Monforte, M. T., Calabro, M. L. HPLC analysis of oleuropein and some flavonoids in leaf and bud of *Olea europaea*. *Il Farmaco*, 1991; 46(6): 803-15.

Pearson, R. B. *Pasteur: Plagiarist, Impostor! The Germ Theory Exploded* (1942). Reprinted Pomeroy, Wash.: National Health Research Association. (See Resources section for information on National Health Research Association.)

_____. *The Dream and Lie of Louis Pasteur*. Collingwood, Australia: Sumeria Press, 1994.

Peck, S. M., and Rosenfeld, H. The effects of hydrogen ion concentration, fatty acids and vitamin C on the growth of fungi. *Journal of Investigative Dermatology*, 1938; 1: 237-65.

Perlman, H. H. Undecylenic acid given orally in psoriasis and neurodermatitis. *Journal of the American Medical Association*, 1949; 139: 444-47.

Peska, J. J., and Bondy, G. S. Alteration of immune function following dietary mycotoxin exposure. *Canadian Journal of Physiology and Pharmacology*, 1990; 68(7): 1009-16.

Qian, G.S., Ross, R.K., Yu, M.C., et al. A follow-up study of urinary markers of aflatoxin exposure and liver cancer risk in Shanghai, People's Republic of China. *Cancer Epidemiology, Biomarkers and Research*, 1994; 3(1):3-10.

Rapaport, S. I. Blood coagulation and its alterations in hemorrhagic and thrombotic disorders. *The Western Journal of Medicine*, 1993; 158: 153.

Ren, A., and Han, X. Dietary factors and esophageal cancer: A case-control study. *Chinese Journal of Epidemiology*, 1991; 12(4): 200-4.

Robey, I.F. et al. Bicarbonate increases tumor pH and inhibits spontaneous metastases. *Cancer Research*, 2009; 69(6): 2260-8.

Rodricks, J. B., Hessiltine, C. W., Mehlman, M. A., eds. *Mycotoxins in Human and Animal Health*. Park Forest South, Ill.: Pathotox Publishers, 1977.

Rosenberg, E. W., Belew, P. W., Skinner, R. B., and Crutcher, N. Response to Crohn's disease and psoriasis. *New England Journal of Medicine*, 1983; 308: 101.

Roum, J.H., Borok, Z., McElvaney, N.G., et al. Glutathione aerosol suppresses lung epithelial surface inflammatory cell-derived oxidants in cystic fi brosis. *Journal of Applied Physiology*, 1999; 87: 438-443.

Saleem, A., et al. Viscoelastic measurement of clot formation: A new test of platelet function. *Annals of Clinical and Laboratory Science*, 1983; 13: 115.

Samiec, P.S., Drews-Botsch, C., Flagg, E.W., et al. Glutathione in human plasma: decline in association with aging, age-related macular degeneration, and diabetes. *Free Radical Biology & Medicine*, 1998; 24:699-704.

Sander, F. F. *The Acid-Base Household of the Human Organism.* 1930

Sandler, M., and Bourne, G. H., eds. *Atherosclerosis and Its Origin.* New York and London: Academic Press, 1963.

Sava, G., Giraldi, T., Mestroni, G., and Zassinovich, G. Antitumor effects of rhodium, iridium, and ruthenium complexes in comparison with cisdichlorodiamino platinum in mice bearing Lewis lung carcinoma. *Chemico-Biological Interactions,* 1983; 45: 1-6.

Schmidinger, M., Budinsky, A.C., Wenzel, C., et al. Glutathione in the prevention of cisplatin induced toxicities. A prospectively randomized pilot trial in patients with head and neck cancer and non small cell lung cancer. *Wien Klin Wochenschr,* 2000; 112: 617-623.

Schwartz, G. J. et al. The lipid messenger OEA links dietary fat intake to satiety. *Cell Metabolism,* October 2008: 8(4):281-288.

Selig, M. S. Mechanisms by which antibiotics increase the incidence and severity of candidiasis and alter the immunological defense. *Bacteriological Review,* 1966; 30: 442-59.

Shaw, C.A., ed. *Glutathione in the Nervous System.* London: Taylor and Francis; 1998.

Shirahata, S., et al: Electrolyzed-Reduced Water Scavenges Active Oxygen Species and Protects DNA from Oxidative Damage, *Biochemical and Biophysical Research Communications,* 234 (1997): 269.

Shook, E. E. *Advanced Treatise in Herbology.* Banning, Calif.: Enos Publishing Co., 1992.

Siegel, L.H. The control of ileostomy and colostomy odors. *Gastroenterology,* 1960; 38: 634-636.

Sies, H. Glutathione and its role in cellular functions. *Free Radical Biology of Medicine,* 1999; 27: 916-921.

Silberberg, J. M., et al. Identification of tissue factor in two human pancreatic cancer cell lines. *Cancer Research,* 1989; 49: 5443.

Silomon, M. Effect of sodium bicarbonate infusion on hepatocyte

Ca2+ overload during resuscitation from hemorrhagic shock. *Resuscitation*, April, 1998; 37 (1): 27-32.

Simonich, M.T. Egner, P.A., Roebuck, B.D., et al. Natural chlorophyll inhibits aflatoxin B1-induced multi-organ carcinogenesis in the rat. *Carcinogenesis*, 2007; 28(6): 1294-1302.

Smith, L.W.. The present status of topical chlorophyll therapy. *New York State Journal of Medicine*, 1955; 55(14): 2041-2050.

Smith, R.G.. Enzymatic debriding agents: an evaluation of the medical literature. *Ostomy Wound Management*, 2008; 54(8): 16-34.

Smyth, J.F., Bowman, A., Perren, T., et al. Glutathione reduces the toxicity and improves quality of life of women diagnosed with ovarian cancer treated with cisplatin: results of a double-blind, randomized trial. *Annals of Oncology*, 1997; 8: 569-573.

Spillert, C. R., et al. Altered coagulability: An aid to selective breast biopsy. *Journal of the National Medical Association*, 1993; 85: 273.

Sprince, H., et al. Protective action of ascorbic acid and sulfur compounds (including N-acetyl cysteine) against toxicity: Implications in alcoholism and smoking. *Agents and Actions*, 1975; 5: 164-73.

Steinmetz, K. A., and Potter, J. D. Food-group consumption and colon cancer in the Adelaide case-control study: Meat, poultry, seafood, dairy foods and eggs. *International Journal of Cancer*, 1993; 53(5): 720-27.

Stephens, D.J. The use of sodium chloride in the treatment of hypopituitarism. *The Journal of Clinical Endocrinology*, 1941; Vol. 1, No. 2 109-112.

Sternberg, P. Jr., Davidson, P.C., Jones, D.P., et al. Protection of retinal pigment epithelium from oxidative injury by glutathione and precursors. *Investigative Opthalmology & Visual Science*, 1993; 34:3661-3668.

Structure, Betina V. Activity relationships among mycotoxins. *Chemico-Biological Interactions*, 1989; 71(2-3): 105-46.

Sudakin, D.L. Dietary aflatoxin exposure and chemoprevention of cancer: a clinical review. *Journal of Toxicology-Clinical Toxicology*, 2003; 41(2): 195-204.

Sugiyama, S., et al. The role of leukotoxin (9, 10-epoxy-12-octadecenoate) in the genesis of coagulation abnormalities. *Life Sciences*, 1988; 43: 221.

Tachino, N., Guo, D., Dashwood, W.M., Yamane, S., Larsen, R., Dashwood, R. Mechanisms of the in vitro antimutagenic action of chlorophyllin against benzo[a]pyrene: studies of enzyme inhibition, molecular complex formation and degradation of the ultimate carcinogen. *Mutation Research*, 1994; 308(2):191-203.

Tallman, M. S., et al. New insights into the pathogenesis of coagulation dysfunction in acute promyelocytic leukemia. *Leukemia and Lymphoma*, 1993; 11: 27.

Topley and Wilson. *Principles of Bacteriology, Virology and Immunity*. Baltimore: Williams & Wilkins, 1984.

Toth, B., and Gannett, P. Carcinogenesis study in mice by 3-methylbutanol methylformylhydrazone of Gyromitra esculenta, in vivo. *Mycopathologia*, 1990; 4(5): 283-88.

Toth, B., Patil, K., Erickson, J., and Kupper, R. False morel mushroom Gyromitra esculenta toxin: N-methyl-N-formylhydrazone carcinogenesis in mice. *Mycopathologia*, 1979; 68(2): 121-28.

Toth, B., Patil, K., Pyssalo, H., Stessman, C., and Gannett, P. Cancer induction in mice by feeding the raw morel mushroom Gyromitra esculenta. *Cancer Research*, 1992; 52(8): 2279-84.

Toth, B., Taylor, J., and Gannett, P. Tumor induction with hexanol methylformylhydrazone of Gyromitra esculenta. *Mycopathologia*, 1991; 115(2): 65-71.

Tranter, H. S., Tassou, S., and Nychas, G. J. The effect of the olive phenolic compound, oleuropein, on growth and enterotoxin B production by Staphylococcus aureus. *Journal of Applied Microbiology*, 1993; 74: 253-59.

Trousseau, A. *Phlegmasia alba dolens Clinique Médicale de l'Hôtel-Dieu de Paris*. London: New Sydenham Society, 1865; 3: 94.

Truss, C. Orian, M.D. *The Missing Diagnosis*. Birmingham, Ala.: The Missing Diagnosis, Inc., 1983.

Uraguchi, K., and Yamazaki, M., eds. *Toxicology, Biochemistry, and Pathology of Mycotoxins*. New York: John Wiley & Son, 1978.

V. Estrella, T. Chen, M. Lloyd, J. Wojtkowiak, H. H. Cornnell, A. Ibrahim-Hashim, K. Bailey, Y. Balagurunathan, J. M. Rothberg, B. F. Sloane, J. Johnson, R. A. Gatenby, R. J. Gillies. Acidity generated by the tumor microenvironment drives local invasion. *Cancer Research*, 2013.

Van Deventer, S. J. H., et al. Intestinal endotoxemia. *Gastroenterology*, 1988; 94(3): 825-31.

Virchow, R. Hypercoagulability: A review of its development, clinical application, and recent progress. *Gesammelte Abhandlungen zur Wissenschäftlichen Medizin*, 1856; 26: 477.

Visioli, F., and Galli, C. Oleuropein protects low density lipoprotein from oxidation. *Life Sciences*, 1994; 55: 1965-71.

Vrijlandt, P. J., Sodium bicarbonate infusion for intoxication with tricyclic antidepressives: recommended in spite of lack of scientific ev dence *Nederlands Tijdschrift voor Geneeskunde*,i Sept., 2001;145(35): 1686-9). Knudsen, K., Epinephrine and sodium bicarbonate independently and additively increase survival in experimental amitriptyline poisoning. *Critical Care Medicine*, Apr 1997; 25(4): 669-74.

Wallach, Joel, BS, DVM, ND *Rare Earths*. Bonita, Calif.: Ma Lan and Double Happiness Publishing Co., 1994.

Weingarten, M., Payson, B. Deodorization of colostomies with chlorophyll. *Revista de Gastroenterologia*, 1951; 18(8): 602-604.

Weir, D., Farley, K.L.. Relative delivery efficiency and convenience of spray and ointment formulations of papain/urea/chlorophyllin enzymatic wound therapies. *Journal of Wound, Ostomy and Continence Nursing*, 2006; 33(5): 482-490.

Westhof, E. *Water and Biological Macromolecules*, CRC Press, Boca Raton, FL: 1993.

White, A., et al., eds. *Principles of Biochemistry*. New York: McGraw-Hill Book Co., 1964.

Wilson, C. L. The alternatively spliced V region contributes to the differential incorporation of plasma and cellular fibronectins into fi brin clots. *Journal of Cell Biology*, 1992; 119: 923.

Witschi, A., Reddy, S., Stofer, B., Lauterburg, B.H. The systemic availability of oral glutathione. *European Journal of Clinical Pharmacology*, 1992; 43:667-669.

Wray, B. B., and O'Steen, J. M. Mycotoxin-producing fungi from house associated with leukemia. *Archived Environmental Health*, 1975; 30: 571-73.

Wray, B. B., Rushing, E. J., Schindel, A., and Boyd, R. C. Suppression of response to phytohemagglutinin in guinea pigs by fungi from a leukemiaassociated house. *Archived Environmental Health*, 1979; 22: 400.

Wylie, T. D., and Morehouse, L. G. *Mycotoxic Fungi, Mycotoxins, Mycotoxicoses: An Encyclopedia Handbook*, Vol. 3.

Yamada, O., et al. Deleterious effects of endotoxins on cultured endothelial cells: An in vitro model of vascular injury. *Inflammation*, 1981; 5: 115.

Yamazaki, H., Fujieda, M., Togashi, M., et al. Effects of the dietary supplements, activated charcoal and copper chlorophyllin, on urinary excretion of trimethylamine in Japanese trimethylaminuria patients. *Life Sciences*, 2004; 74(22): 2739-2747.

Yoshida, S., Kasuga, S. H., Hayashi, N., Ushiroguchi, T., Matsura, H., and Nakagawa, S. Anti-fungal activity of garlic. *Applied and Environmental Microbiology*, 1987; 53(3): 615-17.

Young, R.W., Beregi, J.S. Jr. Use of chlorophyllin in the care of geriatric patients. *Journal of the American Geriatrics Society*, 1980; 28(1): 46-47.

Young, Robert O. *Fermentology and oxidology*. The study of fungus-produced mycotoxic species and the activation of the immune system and release of reactive oxygen toxic species (ROTS) [Self-published]. Alpine, UT: Inner-Light Biological Research Foundation, 1994.

Yun, C.H., Jeong, H.G., Jhoun, J.W., Guengerich, F.P. Non-specifi c inhibition of cytochrome P450 activities by chlorophyllin in human and rat liver microsomes. *Carcinogenesis*, 1995; 16(6):1437-1440.

Zhang, L. Perhydrit and sodium bicarbonate improve maternal gases and acid-base status during the second stage of labor. Department of Obstetrics and Gynecology, Xiangya Hospital, Hunan Medical University, Changsha 410008. Maeda, Y., Perioperative administration of bicarbonate d solution to a patient with mitochondrial encephalomyopathy. *Masui*, Mar 2001; 50(3): 299-303.

Zieve, L., et al. Effect of hepatic failure toxins on liver thymidine kinase activity and ornithine decarboxylase activity after massive necrosis with acetaminophen in the rat. *Journal of Laboratory and Clinical Medicine*, 1985; 106(5): 583-88.

Zwicker, G. M., Carlton, W. W., and Tuite, J. Long-term administration of sterigmatocystin and *Penicillium viridicatum to mice. Food, Cosmetics and Toxicology*, 1974; 12: 491.

ABOUT THE AUTHORS

Robert O. Young, Ph.D., D.Sc., is a nationally renowned microbiologist and nutritionist who speaks to audiences around the world on health and wellness. He holds a degree in microbiology and nutrition and has devoted his life to researching the cause of disease and helping people reclaim their health and well-being. Dr. Young is head of the pH Miracle Living Foundation and has gained national recognition for his research into diabetes, cancer, leukemia, and AIDS. He is a member of the American Society of Microbiologists and the American Naturopathic Association and conducts classes in live blood analysis and the "New Biology." Robert O. Young, Ph.D., D.Sc. provides a dynamic dose of health and nutrition expertise, guaranteed to inform and enlighten. He is the author of The pH Miracle and pH Miracle for Diabetes.

Matt Traverso, is a professional life coach and health consumer advocate who teaches people how to dramatically improve their health naturally, without expensive and potentially dangerous prescription drugs. For the past 15 years he has dedicated his life to finding cutting-edge, breakthrough solutions that are simple yet powerful and have no negative side effects. Today, more than 95% of all chronic disease is caused by diet and lifestyle choices. In his live seminars and conferences, Matt provides the specific tools, skills and coaching necessary to change old habits into new ones for optimal health and vitality. His work has helped thousands of people around the world get off prescription drugs and easily adopt healthy lifestyle choices that make illness and disease simply *vanish*.

Printed in Great Britain
by Amazon